Assessment of a Patient with Lung Disease

Edited by
Jonathan R. Webb, MB, MRCP

Consultant Physician, Brook Hospital and Greenwich
District Hospital, London

Published,
in association with
UPDATE PUBLICATIONS LTD., by

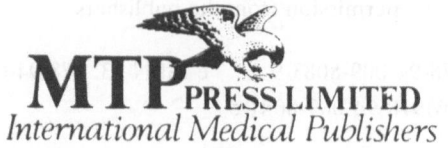

MTP PRESS LIMITED
International Medical Publishers

Published,
in association with
Update Publications Ltd., by

MTP Press Limited
Falcon House
Lancaster, England

Copyright © 1981 MTP Press Limited

Softcover reprint of the hardcover 1st edition 1981

First published 1981

ISBN-13: 978-94-009-8083-9   e-ISBN-13: 978-94-009-8081-5
DOI: 10.1007/978-94-009-8081-5

Contents

List of Contributors

P. D. Buisseret, MB, CH.B, MRCP
Lecturer, Department of Medicine, and Honorary Senior
Lecturer Guy's Hospital Medical School
London

G. M. Cochrane, B.SC, MB, BS, MRCP
Consultant Physician
Guy's Hospital (Teaching) and Lewisham Health District
London

T. W. Higenbottom, B.SC, MB, BS, MRCS, LRCP
Senior Registrar in Thoracic Medicine
Guy's Hospital and Brook Hospital
London

J. G. Kensit, MD, DG, MRCS, LRCP, MRC PATH
Consultant Microbiologist
Queen Mary's Hospital, Sidcup, and Greenwich District
Hospital
London

P. J. Rees, MB, B.CHIR, MRCP
Lecturer
Department of Medicine
Guy's Hospital
London

L. Vogel, MB, BS, MRC.PATH, DCP
Consultant Pathologist and Consultant Cytologist, St
Andrew's Hospital Bow and The London Hospital
London

J. R. Webb, MB, MRCP
Consultant Physician to the Brook Hospital and Greenwich
District Hospital
London

1. The History in Lung Disease

Although the symptoms of respiratory disease may not accurately reflect the degree of functional impairment, a carefully taken clinical history often allows a correct diagnosis to be made (Hampton et al. 1975). The definition of chronic bronchitis is, in fact, based on the clinical history of cough and sputum production. The findings of the history can be evaluated by special investigations.

Major Symptoms

Dyspnoea

Dyspnoea is a feeling that breathing is difficult, laboured or uncomfortable, and there are a number of factors which may lead to the sensation. In some patients it may be difficult to differentiate dyspnoea from pain associated with breathing and, indeed, the limitation of expansion from pleuritic pain may produce a feeling of dyspnoea. Although dyspnoea may be a feature of anxiety it is important to remember that acute dyspnoea is a very distressing situation in itself, quite capable of inducing anxiety in most patients. There are a number of causes of dyspnoea related to the work of breathing, the efficiency of the respiratory muscles and the drive to breathing.

Increased Work of Breathing

The work required for adequate ventilation is increased if there is obstruction to airflow from airway narrowing or if the lungs or the chest wall are abnormally stiff. Both situations increase the mechanical load on breathing and are often associated with dyspnoea.

Neuromuscular Problems

In such conditions as myasthenia gravis and muscular dystrophies the response to the neurological output from the respiratory centre may be inadequate, resulting in a feeling of inability to take in enough air. However, in neuromuscular disorders there may be a paradoxical absence of dyspnoea despite considerable functional impairment. The same situation is found in chronic airflow obstruction associated with CO_2 retention, the 'blue bloater'.

Increased Drive to Breathing

In acidosis and hypoxia there is an increased chemical drive to breathing which stimulates deep, rapid respiration. However, a sensation of dyspnoea may not be prominent if there is not an underlying pulmonary cause for the situation. Dyspnoea may also be found in severe anaemia where the oxygen carrying capacity of the blood is diminished. In chronic airflow obstruction with hypercapnia, the 'blue bloater', the hypercapnia fails to maintain its drive to breathing and dyspnoea is usually absent, despite the hypercapnia and airflow obstruction. In conditions such as pulmonary embolism, pneumonia and pulmonary oedema there seems to be an inappropriately high drive to breathing resulting in hypocapnia. This may be related to stimulation of juxtacapillary, 'J', receptors. Dyspnoea in pneumothorax is probably related to stimulation of a pulmonary deflation reflex. Often a combination of factors is involved in individual cases, for instance in asthma, increased drive, increased load, anxiety and poor muscle function of the diaphragm with overinflation may all be involved.

The pattern of dyspnoea should be assessed. Although orthopnoea is usually described in pulmonary congestion, it is not unusual in chronic airflow obstruction. Shortness of breath waking the patient in the early hours of the morning is often seen in asthma, especially during recovery from an acute attack. Other characteristics of asthma are the day-to-day variation in the severity of the dyspnoea and the relationship to time of year, exercise and environmental factors. Asthma precipitated by extrinsic factors often occurs immediately after exposure but may be delayed for five or six hours, so that asthma induced by exposure at work may only develop after returning home. This makes the relationship more difficult to detect, so that it is important to assess any change in symptoms during weekends or holidays. In chronic airflow obstruction there usually is a slow progression of disability, whereas acute dyspnoea is most often caused by pneumothorax, pulmonary embolism or asthma. The degree of limitation imposed by dyspnoea should be assessed. One system of grading this is shown in Table 1, although it is often best to record the reported exercise tolerance. Although there is not a precise relationship to physiological assessment, the one second forced expiratory volume (FEV_1) is usually less than 0.6 l in patients in grade 5.

Chest Pain

The raw retrosternal pain of acute tracheitis is often associated with virus infections of the upper respiratory tract. Retrosternal pain may be produced by mediastinal lesions such as acute mediastinitis, mediastinal pleurisy or mediastinal tumours. In mediastinal pleurisy the pain is usually continuous rather than typically pleuritic in nature. Occasionally the hilar lymphadenopathy of sarcoidosis is associated with central chest pain.

The commonest chest pain related to the respiratory system is pleuritic pain. This is made worse by the movements of breathing and coughing; it often varies with position and may be related to exercise where respiratory excursions increase. Irritation of the

Table 1. Grading of dyspnoea.

Grade	Description
1	Normal
2	Short of breath on walking up mild hills or stairs
3	Short of breath on walking at a normal pace on level ground
4	Short of breath on walking at own pace on level ground for 100 metres
5	Short of breath on washing, dressing or walking a few paces

diaphragmatic pleura may present as pain in the tip of the shoulder because of the common innervation from the third, fourth and fifth cervical nerves.

Pleuritic pain may occur with rib fractures such as cough fractures which are especially common in patients on long-term corticosteroid therapy. Invasion of the ribs by malignant tumours, however, usually produces a constant, severe, aching pain. Pleuritic pain may be mimicked by epidemic myalgia or Bornholm disease, where breathing is often rapid and shallow to avoid the pain. This condition is distinguished by the tenderness of the overlying muscles and the occurrence in epidemics.

Wheezing

It is important to ask both the patient and any close relative about a history of wheezing, as patients with long-standing wheezing may not consider it relevant. Wheezes have the same significance whether they are heard at the mouth or on listening with the stethoscope. It may be possible to distinguish from the history the loud monophonic wheeze or stridor of tracheal or laryngeal narrowing from the generalized wheezing at many pitches which is a feature of more widespread airway narrowing.

Cough

A cough is the commonest presenting symptom of chest disease. Many smokers regard a morning cough as quite normal and it is not uncommon for patients to admit to sputum production but not to a cough. Coughing may be stimulated by the presence of sputum, foreign bodies, irritant gases, particulate matter or just apposition of bronchial walls. In widespread airflow obstruction it is common to find increased bronchial irritability so that such stimuli as cold air, dry air or increased depth of inspiration produce cough or increased dyspnoea. This is also a feature of the recovery phase from viral infections of the upper respiratory tract. Coughing may also be voluntary and may be a habit or a symptom of anxiety. In asthmatic children a nocturnal cough may be the only presenting symptom noticed by the parents.

Cough is common in association with upper respiratory tract

infections, but requires further investigation if it persists for longer than three weeks. Only relatively large airways are cleared by coughing. Below subsegmental levels airway clearance relies upon the mucociliary escalator carrying mucus or particulate matter up to the level at which coughing becomes effective.

Sputum Production

The volume of sputum, colour, consistency, odour and the time of production should be assessed. It is often difficult to quantify the volume of sputum from the history, but large volumes are typical of bronchiectasis and lung abscesses where the sputum is usually purulent and often foetid from anaerobic infection. In 20 per cent of cases of alveolar cell carcinoma large volumes of pink, frothy sputum are produced.

The sputum may be very viscid in asthma and there may be Curschmann's spirals, which are the casts of small bronchi or the firm brownish plugs which are typical of allergic bronchopulmonary aspergillosis. The expectoration of such casts or plugs may be associated with the relief of acute exacerbations of dyspnoea.

Haemoptysis

Haemoptysis is usually produced in small quantities and massive haemoptysis is an uncommon symptom, although it may be found in bronchiectasis, tuberculosis, mycetomas in old cavities and occasionally with bronchial neoplasms. Haemoptysis is most commonly due to inflamed mucosa in association with acute respiratory tract infections or exacerbations of chronic bronchitis. The initial radiograph is normal in more than half of the patients presenting with haemoptysis and very few extra diagnoses are made on subsequent radiographs taken a month or so later (Poole and Stradling 1964). It is important to investigate haemoptysis fully to rule out tuberculosis and bronchial neoplasms but most series show that neoplasms only make up about four per cent of haemoptyses (Table 2).

In cases of bronchial carcinoma the haemoptysis has usually lasted for longer than two weeks at the time of presentation and usually consists of just blood streaking in the sputum. When the haemoptysis is associated with acute pulmonary symptoms the most common diagnoses are pneumonia and pulmonary infarction, but it must be remembered that pneumonia may be associated with an underlying adenoma or carcinoma.

Other Factors

Smoking History

Smoking is the most important predisposing factor in chronic airflow obstruction and in bronchial carcinoma. The risk of bronchial carcinoma is related to the number and type of cigarettes smoked and smokers of more than 20 cigarettes a day are at a 40 times greater risk than non-smokers (Doll and Hill 1964). The increased carcinoma risk declines slowly for 10 years after stopping smoking. Therefore, details should be recorded of the age of starting and stopping smoking, the amount of tobacco consumed and the average consumption over the smoking period.

Table 2. Causes of haemoptysis.

Cause	Percentage of cases
Upper respiratory tract infection	24
No cause found	21
Bronchitis	17
Bronchiectasis	13
Pneumonia	6
Active tuberculosis	4
Quiescent tuberculosis	6
Cardiovascular	7
Bronchial carcinoma	4

From a review of 324 consecutive cases presenting to a chest clinic (Johnston et al. 1960).

Family History

The most important conditions to ask about in the family history are tuberculosis and atopic conditions. In emphysema the finding of other family members may raise the suspicion of α_1 antitrypsin deficiency. Screening the family may detect pre-symptomatic homozygotes at risk of developing emphysema in whom the onset may be delayed if they can be persuaded not to smoke.

Social History

In asthmatics it is important to ask closely about predisposing factors such as exposure to animal hairs or precipitation of attacks by food or drugs. Many patients do not consider common analgesics or preparations taken for constipation important enough to be mentioned as medications and they should be specifically questioned about such drugs as salicylates and liquid paraffin. Salicylates may precipitate asthma especially in patients with nasal polyposis and intrinsic asthma, and inhaled mineral oils may produce lipoid pneumonia. There is increasing awareness of the association of drugs with a number of respiratory diseases.

Occupational exposure may be relevant to a variety of disorders including asthma, extrinsic allergic alveolitis, pneumoconiosis and neoplasms. In asbestos exposure there is often a long latent period between exposure and development of bronchial carcinoma or mesothelioma. The association may be related to forgotten exposure, such as wartime manufacture of gas masks or servicing of brake linings. It may be related to the husband's occupation if the wife washed her husband's working clothes contaminated with asbestos dust, or even to residence close to an asbestos factory.

2. Examination of the Respiratory System

There are two main parts to the examination of the respiratory system: examination of the chest itself and the assessment of signs outside the chest which relate to respiratory disease. Either part may be examined first. The patient should be reclining comfortably at 45°, stripped to the waist and placed in a good light. The first stage should be general inspection, followed by palpation, percussion and, finally, auscultation. The signs found in common conditions are summarized in Table 3.

Inspection

Any abnormalities in the shape of the chest should be noted. These may be congenital features, such as pectus excavatum, or acquired deformities, such as kyphoscoliosis. Long-standing collapse or fibrosis of the lung may lead to depression of the overlying chest wall; this is most obvious when the upper lobes are involved. Hyperinflation of the lung in asthma or emphysema produces an anteroposterior diameter greater than the lateral diameter. The pattern of breathing should next be observed. The normal respiratory rate is 12 to 16 per minute and not the 20 per minute often recorded in hospital patients.

Abnormal patterns of breathing may give clues to the diagnosis (Table 4), although nervous patients tend to hyperventilate during the examination. Dyspnoeic patients often use their accessory muscles on inspiration and their abdominal muscles on expiration. Any local diminution of chest wall movement is best observed facing the patient from the foot of the bed; reduction in chest wall movement is found with fibrosis, collapse, consolidation, effusion and pneumothorax. Abnormal veins may be present on the chest wall in superior vena caval obstruction. Gynaecomastia may be a sign of bronchial carcinoma or, more commonly, drug therapy such as spironolactone.

Palpation

The position of the mediastinum is assessed from the trachea and the apex beat. The trachea is often best felt with the patient sitting up. With an overinflated chest it may not be possible to feel an apex beat. The impulse of an hypertrophied right ventricle may be felt at the left sternal edge, although with an overinflated chest it is often best felt producing a downward impulse in the epigastrium. In pulmonary hypertension a dilated pulmonary artery may be visible and palpable in the second left interspace. The expansion of the left and right sides of the chest should be compared in upper and lower zones. This is best done with the spread fingers on the chest wall and the thumbs free of the chest, meeting in the midline.

Consolidation allows the transmission of the higher frequency components of speech to the surface and may be felt as increased tactile vocal fremitus (TVF). This is usually easier to detect as increased conduction of voice sounds on auscultation. Pleural friction rubs may sometimes be transmitted to the palpating hand.

Percussion

The information from percussion comes from both the sound and the vibrations felt in the percussed finger. Percussion should start over the clavicles which may be percussed directly and should then proceed down the chest comparing the two sides. The lateral part of the chest must always be examined as well as anterior and posterior surfaces. With overexpansion of the chest the cardiac dullness may be diminished or absent and the top level of the hepatic dullness may be abnormally low. In diaphragmatic paralysis the hepatic dullness may be high and it is sometimes possible to demonstrate that the level does not move with respiration.

Table 3. Signs found in common lung conditions.

Clinical diagnosis	Observation	Movement	Palpation	Percussion
Consolidation		Decreased locally	Mediastinum central ↑ TVF	Dull
Collapse		Decreased locally	Mediastinum towards lesion ↓ TVF	Dull
Fibrosis	Overlying chest wall deformity	Decreased locally	Mediastinum towards lesion ↑ TVF	Dull
Pneumothorax		Decreased locally	Mediastinum may move away from lesion ↓ TVF	↑ Resonance
Pleural effusion		Decreased locally	Mediastinum may move away from lesion ↓ TVF	Stony dull
Chronic bronchitis and emphysema	Prolonged expiration Overexpansion	Decreased excursion		↑ Resonance ↓ Cardiac and hepatic dullness
Asthma	Prolonged expiration Overexpansion	Decreased excursion		↑ Resonance ↓ Cardiac and hepatic dullness
Fibrosing alveolitis	Rapid shallow breathing	Decreased excursion		May be decreased resonance

[1] In upper lobe collapse bronchial breathing may be transmitted from adjacent trachea.

Breath sounds	Voice sounds	Wheezes	Crackles
Bronchial	Bronchophony Whispering pectoriloquy		Pan or late inspiratory
Decreased[1]	Decreased		
Bronchial	Bronchophony Whispering pectoriloquy		Coarse late inspiratory, gravity dependent
Decreased	Decreased		Occasionally click in time with heart beat in shallow left pneumothorax
Decreased	Decreased Aegophony at upper border		May be associated pleural crackles
Prolonged expiration	Decreased	Polyphonic expiratory	Late expiratory and early inspiratory audible at the mouth
Prolonged expiration	Decreased	Polyphonic expiratory or random mono-phonic	Late expiratory and early inspiratory audible at the mouth
		Sequential inspiratory	Fine late inspiratory not conducted to the mouth

Table 4. Patterns of breathing movements.

Locally decreased movement	Fibrosis, collapse, consolidation, effusion, pneumothorax
Rapid shallow breathing	Restrictive ventilatory defect Pleuritic pain
Rapid deep breathing	Metabolic acidosis Brain damage Fever Anxiety
Cheyne–Stokes or periodic breathing	Pulmonary oedema Brain damage Raised intracranial pressure Renal failure
Irregular or 'ataxic' breathing	Brain stem damage Psychogenic
Prolonged inspiration	Laryngeal or tracheal stenosis
Prolonged expiration	Chronic airflow obstruction Asthma
Grunting expiration	Pneumonia
Orthopnoea	Pulmonary oedema Chronic airflow obstruction
Platypnoea (dyspnoea in upright position)	Basal vascular shunts (congenital or portal hypertension)
Inward abdominal movement on inspiration	Severe airflow obstruction Bilateral diaphragm paralysis
Inward thoracic movement on inspiration	Cervical cord transection

Auscultation

The interpretation of lung sounds has been given a sounder physiological basis in recent years by the work of Forgacs (1978). The terminology is simplified by describing added sounds as either wheezes (continuous sounds) or crackles (interrupted sounds). Lung sounds generally have a high frequency range and may be well heard through any efficient stethoscope. However, use of the bell avoids artifactual sounds produced by skin or hair rubbing on the diaphragm.

Breath Sounds

The breath sounds have a frequency range of 200 to 600 Hz (cycles per second) and are heard throughout inspiration and at the beginning of expiration. In bronchial breathing there is little alteration or filtration of the sounds from the large airways. The sounds are similar to those heard over the trachea with an even frequency distribution from 200 to 2000 Hz. They are audible throughout expiration as well as inspiration and are louder than normal breathing. Breath sounds are decreased over hyper-inflated lung, fluid or pneumothorax. However, the size of an effusion or pneumothorax makes little difference to the decrease in sound, which comes largely from reflection of sound at the pleural surfaces where sound conducting properties on the two sides of the pleura change.

Table 5. Crackles.

Clinical diagnosis	Timing	Number	Pitch	Conduction to mouth	Gravity dependence
Pulmonary oedema	Late inspiration	Many	High	Usually no	Yes
Fibrosing alveolitis	Late inspiration	Many	High	No	Yes (until fibrosis severe)
Chronic airflow obstruction	End expiratory and early inspiratory	Few	Low	Yes	No
Pneumonia	Through or late inspiration	Variable	Variable	No	No
Pleurisy	Inspiration, expiration or both	Variable	Usually low	No	May change with position
Bronchiectasis	Inspiration	Variable	'Coarse'	Yes	No

Crackles

Crackles are the result of the sudden opening of closed airways allowing the pressure in the airway above and below the closure to become equal. Nath and Capel (1974) observed the repetitive nature of crackles and related the timing to the underlying pathology. In fibrosing alveolitis and pulmonary oedema the crackles are heard late in inspiration and are usually gravity-dependent, although when the fibrosis is severe the crackles may not change with posture. The pattern of crackles changes on listening at sites a short distance apart. This, together with lack of conduction to the mouth, suggests that these crackles originate in small airways. The late opening of small airways implied from physiological tests lends additional support to this view.

End expiratory and early inspiratory crackles are heard in airflow obstruction. They are probably the result of the passage of boluses of air through intermittently obstructed airways, and are heard at the mouth, with or without the aid of a stethoscope. Other sounds to listen for are pleural crackles (Table 5), clicking sounds in pneumothoraces and a splash with air and fluid in the pleural cavity.

Wheezes (Table 6)

Wheezes are produced in airways whose walls are nearly in contact and oscillate to produce a single note. The pitch is dependent on the nature of the obstruction and the velocity of the gas passing through it, but is not dependent upon the density of the gas or the length and diameter of the adjacent airway. A fixed stenosis caused by a tumour, foreign body or stricture produces a monophonic wheeze often present on inspiration as well as expiration. If the narrowing is in a single lobar bronchus the wheeze may be out of phase with airflow at the mouth. In some situations wheezing may be absent despite severe airway narrowing. In airflow obstruction with carbon dioxide retention ventilation may be reduced to such an extent that airflow is insufficient to cause wheezing. In severe asthma the obstruction may be so far out in the bronchial tree that airflow is too slow to produce wheezing.

Table 6. Wheezes[1]

Wheezing	Associated conditions	Timing	Number of pitches	Audible at mouth
Monophonic	Large airway obstruction	Inspiratory and/or expiratory	One	Yes (stridor)
Polyphonic	Chronic airflow obstruction Asthma	Expiratory	Many	Yes
Random monophonic	Asthma	Inspiratory and expiratory	Few	Yes
Sequential inspiratory	Fibrosing alveolitis	Inspiratory usually late preceding crackles	Few	No

[1] Note that in severe asthma and in hypercapnic respiratory failure there may be a paradoxical absence of wheezing despite severe airway narrowing.

Voice Sounds

Consolidated lung allows the transmission of the higher frequency components of speech to the surface so that the spoken words become recognizable. Whispering is made up of mainly high frequency sounds which are normally filtered out but become audible over consolidated or fibrosed lung. Bronchophony and whispering pectoriloquy have the same implications as bronchial breathing. They may also be heard over a collapsed upper lobe because of the proximity of the trachea, even though the upper lobe bronchus is obstructed. A small amount of pleural fluid filters out the low frequency components of speech and this gives the voice sounds at the upper level of a pleural effusion a peculiar 'bleating' quality known as aegophony.

Other Signs Associated with Respiratory Disease

There are a number of signs which should always be looked for in assessing the patient with respiratory disease. Central cyanosis is best looked for in the buccal mucosa on the inside of the lower lip. It implies the presence of 5 g of desaturated haemoglobin but it is an unreliable sign. In a young asthmatic cyanosis indicates a severe ventilatory defect, which requires emergency treatment. The face may reveal the cyanosed, plethoric complexion of the 'blue bloater' with chronic hypercapnia and often polycythaemia. In superior vena caval obstruction the face appears swollen and cyanosed with watery eyes and distended non-pulsatile neck veins.

The hands should be examined for the bounding pulses, warm extremities and flapping tremor of carbon dioxide retention. Clubbing of the fingers is assessed by looking for an increase of the angle between nail and cuticle above the normal 140°, increased longitudinal and lateral curvature of the nail and sponginess of the nailbed. Clubbing is sometimes associated with hypertrophic pulmonary osteoarthropathy which presents as stiffness, swelling and tenderness at the ends of the long bones, most commonly at the knees, ankles, wrists and elbows. The usual cause is a bronchial neoplasm, although it is found in 50 per cent of cases of pleural fibromas.

The neck should be examined for the jugular pulse, lymphadenopathy and, in the presence of stridor, a thyroid extending retrosternally should be excluded. In right ventricular failure secondary to pulmonary disease there may be a raised jugular venous pressure, peripheral oedema and an enlarged liver. On auscultation a third heart sound may be present at the left sternal edge and occasionally a tricuspid regurgitant murmur. The jugular venous pressure may be difficult to assess in patients with airflow obstruction because of the high positive pleural pressure during expiration.

In the eyes, iridocyclitis is a feature of tuberculosis and sarcoidosis and phlyctenular conjunctivitis may be found in tuberculosis. Examination of the fundi may reveal choroidal tubercles or papilloedema in severe carbon dioxide retention.

If the patient is producing any sputum, this should be examined for blood and purulence. Purulent sputum is usually a sign of infection but may be produced by a large number of eosinophils in asthma.

In the presence of airflow obstruction some objective assessment of the degree of obstruction should be part of the routine examination. This may be done at the bedside by estimating the expiratory peak flow rate. If a peak flow meter is not available the forced expiratory time can be estimated; more than five seconds to expel the full vital capacity being abnormal. The maximum distance walked in a set time, usually 12 minutes, is a useful assessment of the degree of limitation imposed by the disease. In acute asthma a check can be kept on the amount of pulsus paradoxus measured by a sphygmomanometer. These measurements can be repeated to keep a check on the progress of the condition.

The Chest Radiograph

The chest radiograph is established as an essential part of the assessment of patients with respiratory disease. The usual view is the posteroanterior (PA) view, but a lateral film is generally necessary for precise anatomical localization. It also shows up such areas as the retrosternal and retrocardiac areas which are not visible on routine PA films. The use of a high kilovoltage technique (135 to 150 kV peak) is now becoming more widespread. This provides significantly better definition of the details of the lung fields with a decreased dose of radiation to the lungs. However, the bones are less clearly seen and conventional techniques should be used if these are important.

The chest radiograph provides information about the whole chest and the inexperienced observer should go through a mental checklist of soft tissue, bones, trachea and mediastinum, heart, diaphragm, hila, fissures, and pleura on each occasion. Although the radiograph gives anatomical information which is necessary to define the precise extent of any lesion which may be suspected on clinical examination, it is not a functional assessment. Such conditions as emphysema, chronic bronchitis and asthma may produce little or no abnormality on the chest radiograph even at a time when they are clinically quite severe. Acute changes in these diseases may not be reflected in the radiograph other than in the hyperinflation often associated with exacerbations of airflow obstruction. However, the chest radiograph is very useful in following the course of anatomical lesions such as localized opacities.

The management of patients who present with abnormal radiographs may be greatly simplified if old films are available. Any such valuable information should be vigorously pursued. Patients in hospital sometimes have radiographs repeated at unnecessarily frequent intervals. For instance, in a patient with pneumonia who is showing the expected clinical response to antibiotics there is no indication to repeat the radiograph in less than a week. The changes in pneumonia may be very slow to clear and this usually raises the suspicion of an underlying malignancy. In Boyd's series of 64 cases of poorly resolving pneumonia only one patient turned out to have a pulmonary neoplasm (Boyd 1975). In the others, radiological clearing continued for up to six months and apparently permanent changes remained in 50 patients.

Tomography is a useful technique in demonstrating cavitation and calcification and in assessing hilar lesions. It may be valuable in the diagnosis by demonstrating such features as satellite lesions in tuberculosis or the presence of feeding vessels in arteriovenous malformations. Computerized axial tomography is now proving useful in the assessment of mediastinal lesions and further developments will probably widen its scope in respiratory disease.

3. Microbiological Investigation of Lung Disease

Efficient and effective use of the laboratory demands a clear idea of the value and limitations of laboratory investigations in chest disease. In some conditions why perform any tests at all? For example, acute exacerbations of chronic bronchitis are treated successfully in general practice, almost invariably without laboratory examination of sputum.

There are occasions when rational therapy can be based only on laboratory results. Chest infections requiring antimicrobial therapy in children with cystic fibrosis are usually caused by *Haemophilus influenzae*, *Staphylococcus aureus* or *Pseudomonas aeruginosa*. Identification of the causative organism is required since different antibiotics must be used against them.

Isolation of patients to prevent cross-infection may depend on a precise microbiological diagnosis. For example, cases of 'open' tuberculosis with acid fast bacilli seen in sputum smears; pneumonias caused by *Staphylococcus aureus* with widespread dissemination of the organism; and infections with respiratory syncytial virus which is particularly dangerous to infants. Laboratories may assist in the investigation of the epidemiology of infections. Many viral infections have been carefully studied, unfortunately with as yet little practical application. Of more immediate value is the monitoring of the prevalence of resistance to antibiotics of an organism such as *Haemophilus influenzae*, allowing more rational blind therapy in infections associated with this organism. As a final example the prevalence of the recently recognized 'Legionnaire's disease' is under investigation.

Sputum Examination in Bacterial Infections

Collection

The normal respiratory tract below the larynx is sterile, though patients with chronic bronchitis may harbour non-capsulate haemophili. Expectorated sputum passes through the throat and mouth areas with a rich and varied flora which includes almost all the organisms capable of causing chest infections. Thus the isolation of a potential pathogen from such material may be irrelevant. Collection techniques that minimize oral contamination are essential. The patient should be asked to wash out his mouth, if possible, with sterile water and then to cough up a sample of sputum into a sterile container. Mouthwash may be bactericidal and must not be used before specimen collection.

Specimens are best collected in the early morning and some patients are incapable of producing sputum for the rest of the day. Amateur physiotherapy and hanging the patient over the side of the bed are both very helpful. The assistance of a physiotherapist proper is always useful. A good specimen is mucoid or purulent with minimal salivary contamination, and no food particles. Patients who cannot produce sputum either have none or are drowning in their own secretions. In the former case there is no point in sending saliva for examination and in the latter they need suction, which will provide the required specimen.

Other Collection Methods: Suction via Endotracheal Tubes

It can be shown that many patients with endotracheal tubes in situ rapidly develop bronchial flora similar to mouth flora. Examination of specimens and interpretation of results are similar to those for expectorated sputum.

Bronchoscopy

Material from the throat is carried on the instrument into the bronchi even with the best technique. Culture will usually show scanty oral flora even when other techniques demonstrate sterile bronchial secretions.

By-passing the Larynx—Transtracheal Aspiration

After skin infiltration with local anaesthetic the operator passes a needle into the trachea through the cricothyroid membrane and threads a plastic catheter down into the bronchi. Any secretions present are then aspirated. This method is more popular in the USA than the UK, and is particularly useful in diagnosis of anaerobic lung infections where the results of expectorated sputum culture may be actively misleading. However, the method does require expertise and is often frightening to the patient.

Tracheostomy

At first site collection of sputum via the tracheostomy seems to have the advantages of transtracheal aspiration without the disadvantages. However, the stoma of a tracheostomy is rapidly colonized by various Gram negative bacilli (GNBs) and aspiration of bronchial secretions for laboratory examination frequently results in contamination of specimens. Furthermore, pharyngeal secretions may enter bronchi as described with endotracheal tubes. Results of culture must again be interpreted with care.

Lung Aspiration

This is the most direct method of diagnosis but is only a research tool at present. Complications are few in expert hands.

Transport

Ideally sputum specimens should be examined immediately since some pathogens die relatively quickly and some of the hardier contaminating organisms may multiply at room temperature. However, it is generally satisfactory to examine the specimen within three to four hours of collection, and if a longer delay is going to occur, refrigeration for up to 24 hours is acceptable.

The Organisms

Pneumococci *(Streptococcus pneumoniae)*

Pneumococci are Gram positive cocci, classically seen as diplococci (Plate 1). Until recently all strains were penicillin-sensitive, but moderately resistant strains now occur worldwide, although they are still rare, and in the UK these strains are very rare. The organism is commonly found in the throat flora and may cause lobar and bronchopneumonia.

Haemophilus influenzae

These Gram negative coccobacilli are found in many throats as non-capsulate strains and are part of the normal flora at this site. They are rarely pathogenic other than in acute exacerbations of chronic bronchitis (Plate 2). Capsulate forms are less common, but may give rise to meningitis, epiglottitis and very rarely true Haemophilus pneumonia. Recent work suggests that capsulate strains may be involved in chest infections more commonly than hitherto thought. Ampicillin resistance is uncommon—approximately 1.5 per cent of strains isolated in the UK.

Staphylococcus aureus

Staphylococcus aureus is a Gram positive coccus, and is classically seen in clusters in sputum Gram stains (Plate 3). These bacteria are a common cause of pneumonia in patients with cystic fibrosis, and of bacterial pneumonia in influenza and following other viral illnesses. It should be remembered that most strains isolated from patients both in and out of hospital are resistant to benzylpenicillin.

Klebsiella pneumoniae (Friedlander's bacillus)

Klebsiella pneumoniae is a rare cause of lobar pneumonia. Classical Friedlander's pneumonia may be caused by any of several capsule types in the genus *Klebsiella*. Most isolates are secondary invaders and of low pathogenicity.

Pseudomonas aeruginosa

Isolation of *Pseudomonas aeruginosa* from the lower respiratory tract has been associated with four syndromes:

1. Simple colonization, which does not require therapy.
2. Indirect pathogenicity by destroying antibiotics, e.g. ampicillin

and cotrimoxazole and allowing other, otherwise sensitive, pathogens to flourish (e.g. *H. influenzae*).

3. Pathogen in chronic infection, e.g. cystic fibrosis or bronchiectasis from any cause. The bacteria are usually present as a mucoid colonial type and are very difficult to eliminate with therapy.

4. Acute infection caused by *Pseudomonas pneumonia*, which is very rare, very acute, usually lethal and often indicates underlying immune abnormalities.

Other Gram Negative Bacteria

Other GNBs, e.g. *E. coli*, *Citrobacter* sp., *Serratia* sp. are essentially secondary invaders and are not commonly pathogenic. They are isolated particularly from sputum produced by patients already on antibiotics.

Effect of Antibiotic Therapy

After one dose of an antibiotic it may be impossible to culture pneumococci or haemophili from the sputum. A Gram stain may still indicate their pathogenic role. If sputum is to be cultured, the specimens should be obtained before antimicrobial therapy. Negative cultures during therapy do not exclude the presence of the above pathogens. When patients are receiving antimicrobial therapy their normal oral flora is largely replaced by Gram negative bacilli such as *E. coli* and *Klebsiella* sp. Consequently, these organisms are often isolated on culture during therapy; they should not be assumed to be pathogens.

Other evidence, such as the clinical condition of the patient, chest radiograph findings, white cell count and sputum Gram film need to be considered before a diagnosis of Gram negative pneumonia is made. Many people taking antibiotics will produce Gram negative bacilli in their sputum, but do not necessarily have pneumonia. Furthermore, failing to culture pneumococci or haemophili does not necessarily mean that they are not still active in the patient.

Antigen Detection

Poor cultural results, partly caused by prior antibiotic therapy, have led some investigators to look for pneumococcal antigen in sputum by immunoelectrophoresis. This investigation is sometimes valuable but it is unclear whether it is a generally useful diagnostic tool. In general, if the organism can be isolated then antigen is detectable, but antigen may be detectable when no pneumococci are grown. The incidence of the latter occurrence varies widely, but there is no doubt that once antibiotics have been given antigen detection is vastly superior to sputum culture.

Tuberculosis

Many of the above comments on sputum collection are applicable in the diagnosis of pulmonary tuberculosis. However, *Mycobacterium tuberculosis* is not a normal inhabitant of the upper respiratory tract, and therefore its isolation is always significant.

Microscopy

The laboratory diagnosis of tuberculosis hinges on sputum staining (usually with Ziehl–Nielson (ZN) stain) and subsequent culture. Mycobacteria are difficult to stain, but once stained are difficult to decolorize. Smears of sputum are stained with hot carbol fuchsin and then decolorized with acid or acid–alcohol. Mycobacteria are the only organisms to resist decolorization. The slide is then counterstained with methylene blue. Mycobacteria appear as red bacilli on a blue background (Plate 4). Auramine–phenol staining may be used instead of carbol fuchsin, the tubercle bacilli fluorescing under UV light. This allows rapid screening of specimens, but positive results should be checked by ZN staining.

Culture must never be omitted. First, it confirms a positive by staining and allows identification of the organism and sensitivity testing. Second, ZN staining is a relatively insensitive technique for diagnosing pulmonary tuberculosis. It has been estimated that approximately 50,000 organisms/ml sputum must be present before scanty acid fast bacilli (AFB) are seen on slides. Culture allows detection of only a very few organisms per ml of sputum. Third, organisms seen on smears may be non-viable in patients already on therapy.

Culture

Mycobacterium tuberculosis grows slowly, cultures taking from 3 to 16 or more weeks to become positive. Contaminating respiratory tract flora grows much more quickly than this and the specimen must be treated to eliminate these. Such treatment depends on the relative insensitivity of Mycobacteria to alkali which rapidly kills non-mycobacteria. The specimen is neutralized and cultured on suitable solid media. Guinea-pig inoculation is rarely, if ever, used, largely because the sensitivity in detecting mycobacteria is no better than with currently available artificial media.

Mycobacteria other than *Mycobacterium tuberculosis* are rarely involved in lung infections. *Mycobacterium kansasii* is the most commonly isolated member of this group and appears to cause one to two per cent of all cases of pulmonary tuberculosis. Repeat isolates of the same species are necessary to confirm their significance as pathogens, rather than incidental contaminates.

Viral Infections

Viral respiratory tract infections are common and it is impossible and unnecessary to investigate them all. However, in some clinical situations laboratory investigations are clearly warranted.

Therapy of some viral infections is now possible, e.g. herpes simplex lesions may be treated with idoxuridine, and the advent of more relatively non-toxic antiviral agents may necessitate a precise aetiological diagnosis in many viral illnesses. However, no drugs are yet available to treat viral respiratory infections, the vast majority of which are in any case trivial and self-limiting.

Studies of respiratory syncytial virus in babies have shown that hospital cross-infection among these children is common and that the resulting illness may be severe. It is thus worth making the diagnosis in order to isolate the infected patients. A precise diagnosis may be essential in the management of contacts of some virus diseases (e.g. rubella), but this is not applicable to any of the respiratory virus infections.

The cost of virological tests, particularly virus culture, is considerable and clinicians requesting tests should consider the value of the result obtained and be able to justify the expense and work required to produce it.

Culture

Culture has the advantages of being the most sensitive diagnostic method available and of providing direct evidence of the presence of virus. However, it is also slow, taking from a few days to a few weeks to produce evidence of virus growth, and it is an expensive system. Most viruses infect the whole of, rather than a part of, the respiratory tract, though they may produce symptoms confined to particular parts only. Consequently any secretions may contain viruses and it is usual to culture throat swabs, though pernasal aspirates and sputum may also be suitable. Swabs should be taken into a suitable transport medium, many viruses being highly labile outside the body.

Antigen Detection by Fluorescence

This method has been useful in the rapid diagnosis of respiratory syncytial virus infection in children. Nasal secretions are aspirated and smeared onto slides which are stained with a fluoroscein-labelled specific antibody. Infected cells are fluorescent in UV light. The method is very rapid, but does rely on good specimens, preferably collected by the laboratory, high titre and specific antisera and an experienced microscopist. The method clearly has great potential, given suitable antisera.

Serology

Virus infection almost always leads to the production of serum antibodies and a fourfold rise in antibody titre between acute and convalescent sera is taken to indicate recent infection. If serum taken in the acute phase of the illness is unavailable, then diagnosis rests on the finding of a single high titre of antibody. Such titres indicate only recent or past infection and should be interpreted with care.

Other Microbial Agents

Mycoplasma pneumoniae, Coxiella burneti, Chlamydia psittaci

All these organisms may produce the clinical picture of 'primary atypical pneumonia'. They may be cultured from respiratory tract secretions, a time-consuming and difficult procedure. Diagnosis rests on serological evidence, preferably a rising antibody titre.

Pneumocystis carinii

Infection with *Pneumocystis carinii* usually presents in the immunosuppressed patient. Laboratory diagnosis depends on demonstration of the organism in lung obtained by drill biopsy or open biopsy at a limited thoracotomy. Examination of sputum is not useful. In view of the problems of obtaining suitable material for the laboratory a clinical diagnosis is frequently made and confirmed by the rapid response to co-trimoxazole therapy.

Aspergillus fumigatus and *A. niger*

Aspergillus fumigatus and *A. niger* may colonize lung cavities (tuberculous or carcinomatous), forming aspergillomata. These organisms are very rarely invasive though they can produce systemic infection in the immunosuppressed patient. They may be cultured from sputum, and precipitins are frequently demonstrable in serum.

Candida albicans

Candida albicans is a yeast found in small numbers as part of the normal mouth flora. It tends to overgrow when a patient is on antibiotic therapy, and may be grown in large numbers in sputum specimens. It is rarely pathogenic in the lung.

4. Lung Function Tests

Lung function tests are of value in defining disease quantitatively from a functional aspect and in monitoring effects of treatment, and they are becoming increasingly useful in the detection of industrial lung diseases and in monitoring the physiology of ageing. The main function of the lungs is to exchange carbon dioxide and oxygen with pulmonary capillary blood. This requires an efficient set of bellows, conducting airways and gas exchange mechanisms. Tests of lung function in routine use include the following:

1. The volume of gas in the lungs and its various subdivisions (static lung volumes).

2. The ability of the lungs to conduct gas out of the chest as rapidly as possible (the forced expiratory manoeuvre).

3. The ability of the lungs to transfer carbon monoxide (CO) from outside the body into the pulmonary capillary blood (the CO transfer test).

4. The ability of the lungs to maintain normal levels of $P\text{a}_{CO_2}$, $P\text{a}_{O_2}$ and (H^+) (see Chapter 5).

Tests of Lung Function

Static Lung Volumes

Lung function tests date back to Hutchinson's classical experiments of measuring the vital capacity with a spirometer (Hutchinson 1846). Figure 1 shows the most commonly used division of lung volumes. The vital capacity and its subdivisions are easily measured using a spirometer. The measurement of absolute lung volumes requires more sophisticated equipment. There are two methods used in measuring the absolute lung volumes, total lung capacity (TLC) and residual volume (RV): a dilution method using helium and a plethysmographic method (Dubois et al. 1956).

Helium Dilution Method

The helium dilution method involves the subject breathing in and out of a bag of known volume containing a known concentration of helium until equilibration has taken place with the gas in the lungs. The point in the patient's vital capacity at which he enters the circuit containing the helium mixture is known and so the volume of gas in the lungs can be calculated (see Figure 2). This calculation makes the assumption that helium, being an inert and highly insoluble gas, will not be absorbed into the blood or tissue

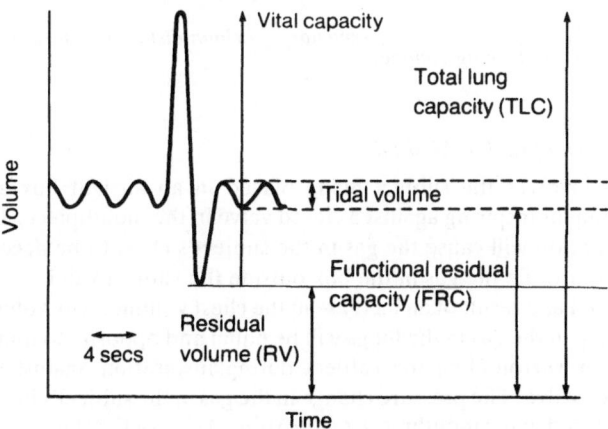

Figure 1. *Spirogram tracing showing lung volumes.*

fluids of the lungs. This method is prolonged for patients with airflow obstruction since equilibration of the helium with the gas in the lungs may take more than 20 minutes in severe airflow obstruction due to slow mixing of the gases.

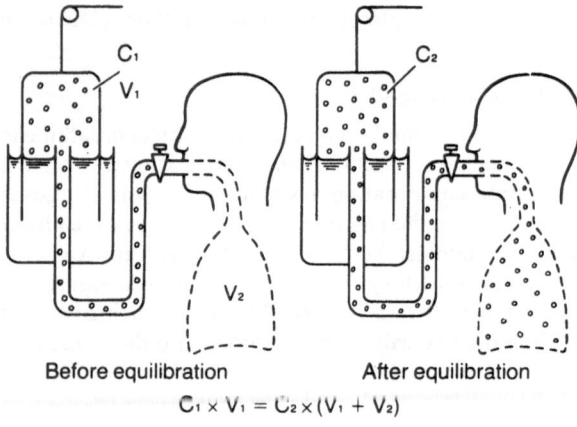

Before equilibration　　　　After equilibration

$$C_1 \times V_1 = C_2 \times (V_1 + V_2)$$

Figure 2. *Diagrammatic representation of helium distribution method of measuring static lung volumes.*

Plethysmographic Method

This involves the subject being placed in an airtight box and panting or inspiring against a closed valve in the mouthpiece. The inspiration will cause the gas in the subject's chest to be decompressed while the gas in the box outside the subject will be compressed as a result of an increase in the chest volume. Any volume change in the gas in the lungs will be equal and opposite to that in the air surrounding the subject during inspiration against the closed valve. The pressure change in the gas in the subject's lung is measured in the mouthpiece on the subject side of the shutter (see Figure 3). This method is quick and accurate and is not affected by airways obstruction, but it does require expensive equipment.

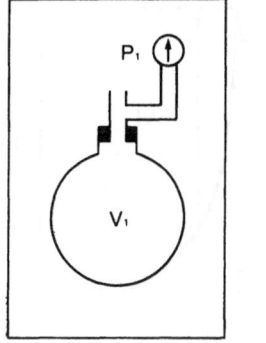 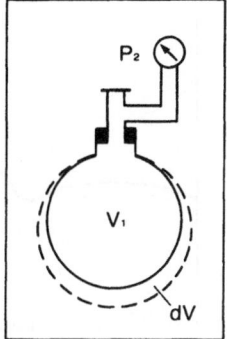

$$P_1 \times V_1 = P_2 \times (V_1 + dV)$$

Figure 3. *Plethysmographic method of measuring static lung volumes. The patient's lungs are represented by the flask volume V. On the right of the diagram inspiration against a closed valve increases the volume to V + dv and reduces the pressure to P_2. In essence, Boyle's Law states that the product of the original pressure and volume of a gas is equal to the product of the new volume and pressure after decompression (or compression). The volume V can be calculated from the above equation.*

The Forced Expiratory Manoeuvre

The forced expiratory manoeuvre involves the subject taking a maximum inspiration and then forcibly exhaling his vital capacity as rapidly as possible down to residual volume. The measurements taken most commonly during this manoeuvre are the forced vital capacity (FVC) and the forced expiratory volume in one second (FEV_1) which requires a measurement of exhaled volume on the vertical axis against time in seconds on the horizontal axis (see Figure 4). A more recent method used is the plotting of the flow rate of gas leaving the mouth on the vertical axis against the exhaled volume on the horizontal axis—the flow volume curve. A useful measurement taken during the manoeuvre is the peak expiratory flow. This measurement is normally made as a separate manoeuvre on a Wright's peak flow meter.

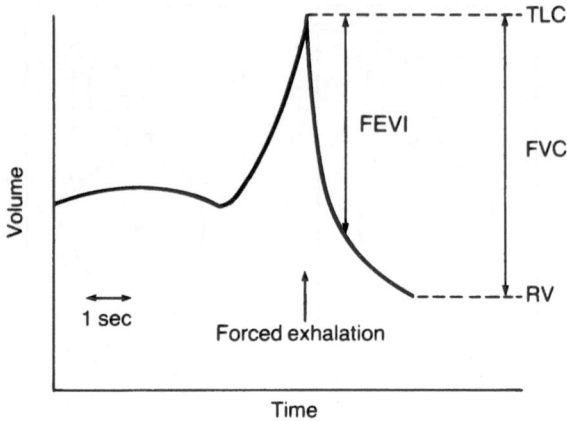

Figure 4. *Spirogram tracing of forced expiratory manoeuvre.*

The Carbon Monoxide Transfer Test ($T_L$co)

This test measures the ability of the lung to transfer or conduct CO from the mouth to the pulmonary capillary blood. It is helpful to think in terms of CO conductance, because the conductance can be substituted into the well-known Ohm's law equation:

$$\text{Resistance} = \frac{\text{Driving pressure}}{\text{Flow}}$$

$$\text{Conductance} = \frac{\text{Flow}}{\text{Driving pressure}} \quad \text{(since resistance} = 1/\text{conductance)}$$

$$\text{CO transfer or conductance} = \frac{\text{Amount of CO transferred per minute from alveolar gas to pulmonary capillary blood}}{\text{Mean alveolar CO pressure} - \text{mean pulmonary capillary CO pressure}}$$

Single Breath Test

The simplest and most commonly used method of determining the CO transfer factor is the modified single breath test (Forster et al. 1955). The subject inhales from residual volume to TLC, a gas containing a very small known concentration of CO and a known concentration of helium. The breath is held for 10 seconds and then completely exhaled (see Figure 5). The concentration of CO and helium in the exhaled alveolar gas sample is then measured. The CO will have diffused into the pulmonary capillary blood during breath-holding and the helium will have been merely diluted by the residual volume of gas in the lungs prior to the inspiration of test gas.

The residual volume can be calculated by using the dilution principle already explained and so the total CO lost from the system during breath-holding and the CO concentration in the aveolar gas at the beginning of breath-holding can be calculated. The concentration of CO in the alveolar gas at the end of breath-holding can be measured directly from the exhaled alveolar gas sample. The mean concentration of CO in the alveolar gas can be

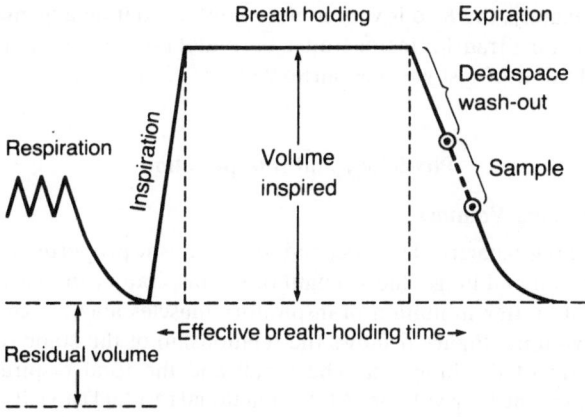

Figure 5. *Modified single breath test for measuring CO transfer (see text).*

calculated using the appropriate equation since the fall in CO concentration during breath-holding is exponential.

We now have all the values necessary to calculate the CO transfer; the mean pulmonary capillary CO concentration can be taken as zero because the affinity of haemoglobin for CO is so vast that the very small quantities of CO transferred to pulmonary capillary blood are almost immediately removed from solution and chemically bound to the haemoglobin. The 'alveolar volume' calculated using the helium dilution technique during the single breath method for $T_L co$ is normally quoted in any value given for the $T_L co$. This is the same value as TLC measured using a body plethysmograph or helium dilution method in normal people.

In patients with airflow obstruction or uneven ventilation the distribution of helium and CO during the 10-second breath-holding will not be complete and so the values obtained for the alveolar volume and the $T_L co$ will drop. The transfer factor is often expressed per litre of alveolar volume and is then referred to as the diffusion constant $K co$ ($K co = T_L co$/alveolar volume). In patients with airflow obstruction, the $T_L co$ and alveolar volume will drop because of incomplete distribution of CO and helium. Although the $T_L co$ and alveolar volume do not drop proportionately, the $K co$ is very useful in differentiating a 'genuine' drop in lung transfer factor from a drop that is secondary to poor distribution of test gas, e.g. airflow obstruction.

Physiology and Interpretation

Static Lung Volumes

Total lung capacity (TLC) depends on the elastic properties of the chest wall and lungs, the strength of the inspiratory muscles and possible reflex inhibition of inspiratory muscles above a certain lung volume. Figure 6 shows the relationship of the static recoil pressure of the lungs, the chest wall and the total respiratory system to the lung volume. At the functional residual capacity, the elastic recoil of the lungs tending to deflate the lungs is equal and opposite to that of the chest wall attempting to spring open.

Changes in Elastic Recoil due to Disease

Diseases that decrease the elastic recoil of the lung, such as emphysema, will cause an increase in TLC, because the elastic recoil of the total respiratory system at any given lung volume will have decreased and, presuming no change in the inspiratory muscle power, the TLC will increase. During an acute attack of asthma the TLC will increase by as much as 1.5 l within a few minutes (Peress et al. 1976), which is remarkable since this means that there is a rapid change in one or a combination of the factors determining TLC.

Reduction in TLC occurs in association with collapse and consolidation. It also occurs in patients with a restrictive defect, which can be considered to be a non-obstructive form of ventilatory defect in which there is a restriction in expansion of the thorax

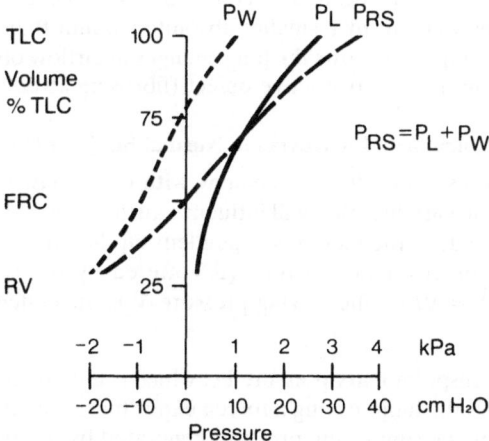

Figure 6. *Relationship of static recoil pressure of the lungs, the chest wall and the total respiratory system to the lung volume. P_W = recoil pressure of chest wall (dotted line), P_L = recoil pressure of the lung (solid line), P_{RS} = recoil pressure of the respiratory system ($P_W + P_L = P_{RS}$).*

due to changes in the lungs (diffuse pulmonary fibrosis) or the chest wall (ankylosing spondylitis or kyphoscoliosis). The reason for the change in both these forms of restrictive defect is decreased compliance (increased stiffness) of the lungs and chest wall, respectively. This results in an increased elastic recoil of the total respiratory system at any given lung volume with a consequent reduction in TLC.

Changes in Vital Capacity due to Disease

In diseases that cause an increase in TLC (emphysema and asthma) VC is usually reduced since there is an increase in the residual volume which is greater in absolute terms than the increase in TLC. In other forms of airflow obstruction (e.g. chronic obstructive bronchitis) the TLC may be within normal limits but the VC will again be reduced as a result of an increase in RV. This can be expressed as an increase in the RV/TLC ratio. In diseases that cause a decrease in TLC (diffuse pulmonary fibrosis) there is also an associated decrease in VC. The RV is often reduced as well but by a smaller absolute amount than the TLC reduction. Figure 7 shows the lung changes in airflow obstruction (emphysema) and a restrictive defect (fibrosing alveolitis).

Forced Expiratory Manoeuvres in Normal Subjects (Pride 1971)

It is again useful to draw an analogy with Ohm's law when considering the variables that will influence airflow rates. Airflow (I) from alveolus to the mouth is dependent on the driving pressure (V) and the resistance to flow (R) offered by the conducting airways: $I = V/R$. The driving pressure V is dependent on two factors:

1. The transpulmonary pressure P_T, which is the pressure generated across the lungs during a forced expiratory manoeuvre. This pressure is the sum of the pressure generated by the respiratory muscles and the elastic recoil of the chest wall.

2. The elastic recoil pressure of the lungs P_L. The elastic recoil of the lungs is responsible for 'collapsing' or emptying the alveoli, i.e. driving air towards the mouth, and it is also responsible for hold-

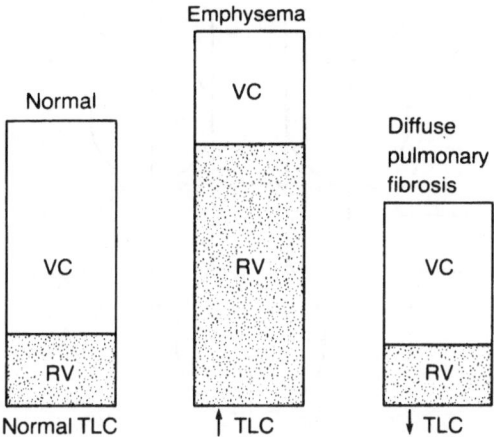

Figure 7. *Comparative lung volume changes in emphysema and diffuse pulmonary fibrosis.*

ing the airways open (see Figure 8).

The resistance of the conducting airways during a forced expiratory manoeuvre is dependent on the diameter of the airways and the phenomenon of dynamic compression. In Figure 9a the forces acting on the lung during conditions of no flow are shown. (The chest wall is represented by a cylinder; the force generated by the chest wall by the piston. The alveoli are represented by a circle and the conducting airways by a tube.) In Figure 9b the forces generated during a forced expiration are shown. The lung volume and hence the elastic recoil pressure are the same as in Figure 9a, and the only change is in P_T. There will now be a pressure gradient from the alveolus to the mouth end of the tube. A transbronchial pressure gradient tending to collapse the airways will build up as the mouth is approached.

This phenomenon of dynamic compression occurs in normal people during a forced expiratory manoeuvre throughout approximately the lower 75 per cent of the vital capacity and can

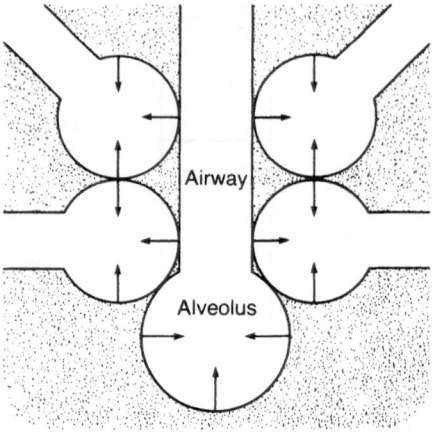

Figure 8. *Elastic recoil forces of lungs acting to collapse the alveoli and keep airways open.*

be seen during bronchoscopy under local anaesthetic, when the flexible posterior membrane of the bronchi collapses inwards on coughing. When dynamic compression occurs, maximum expiratory flow rates become independent of maximum effort, because any increase in driving pressure is met by an equal increase in the resistance to flow.

This was first demonstrated by Fry and Hyatt (1960) who introduced isovolume pressure flow curves. These curves are constructed by measuring the flow rates of gas leaving the mouth at varying driving pressures (P_{alv}) all carried out at the same lung volume. An isovolume pressure flow curve can be constructed at different lung volumes (see Figure 10, right hand side). Using the vertical axis (flow) as common to both sides of the diagram it is possible to construct a flow volume curve using the horizontal axis on the left side of the diagram to represent volume. The isovolume pressure flow curves plateau, except at high lung volume, and so the flow volume curve is effort-independent at these points when the isovolume pressure curves reach a plateau. The term effort-

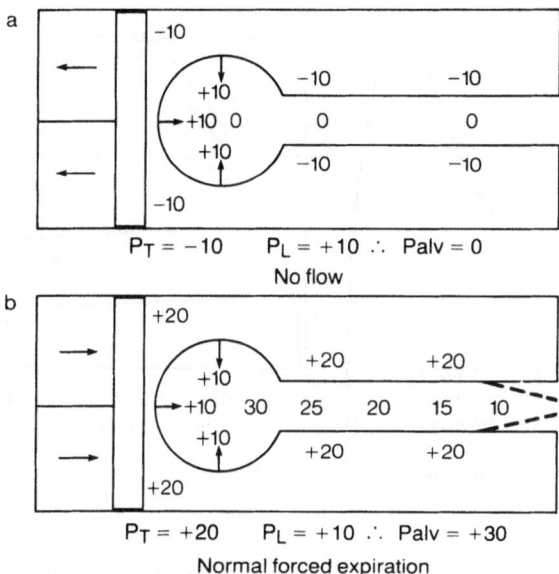

Figure 9. *Conditions during no flow (a) and a forced expiration (b). The alveolar pressure P_{alv} is equal to the sum of the elastic recoil P_L and the transpulmonary pressure P_T, i.e. $P_L + P_T = P_{alv}$ (see text for explanation).*

independence means that the amount of expiratory effort required to produce a maximum flow rate is not maximal, the implication being that the reproducibility of the effort-independent part of the curve will be greater than that for the effort-dependent part of the curve. The commonly used measurement of peak expiratory flow rate (PEFR) can be seen to be effort-dependent.

Forced Expiratory Manoeuvre in Patients with Airflow Obstruction

Patients with airflow obstruction empty their lungs more slowly than normal subjects during a forced expiration. This means that

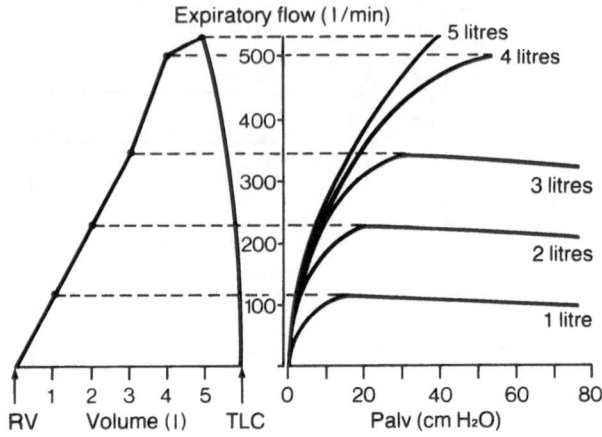

Figure 10. *Flow volume curve (see text).*

the flow rate of gas leaving the mouth at any given lung volume must be reduced. Flow rate has already been shown to be dependent on the driving pressure P_{alv} and the resistance of the conducting airways. Theoretically, the flow rate could be reduced in the following ways:

1. Decreasing P_{alv}. In practice the commonest way for this to occur is by loss of elastic recoil P_L, as seen in emphysema. Theoretically, P_T could be reduced by disease of the chest wall or respiratory muscles, but it is probable that this does not often constitute a clinical problem in patients with airflow obstruction.

2. Increasing resistance in the conducting airways. This can occur by narrowing of the airways which is thought to be the main factor in chronic obstructive bronchitis and asthma. It can also occur as a result of increased 'collapsibility' of the conducting airways, either as a result of intrinsic physical changes in the bronchial walls themselves or as a result of loss of elastic recoil of the lung tending to keep the airways open.

Assessment of Expiratory Flow Limitation

FEV_1 and the ratio of FEV_1 to FVC and PEFR are the most commonly used methods of assessing expiratory flow limitation. Flow rates over the lower half of the vital capacity are said to reflect events occurring in the small airways for the following reasons. The elastic recoil of the lung decreases from TLC to RV. The point in the airways where dynamic compression of the airways occurs during a forced expiratory manoeuvre is dependent primarily on the elastic recoil of the lung: the greater the lung recoil the nearer the mouth dynamic compression occurs. As RV is approached, the point at which dynamic compression occurs will move towards the alveoli. The flow rates achieved at the mouth are dependent on the driving pressure and resistance of the airways upstream (on the alveolar side) of these points where dynamic compression begins to occur (the so-called equal pressure points, EPP, where pressure on the outside of the airway is equal to the pressure on the inside). The resistance to the flow offered by the airways downstream from these EPP is not a flow-limiting factor, and so flow is dependent on the resistance of the upstream segment which over the lower half of the VC tends to be in smaller airways.

Figure 11 shows the flow volume curves in various diseases. The points to notice are that in emphysema the flow rates are markedly reduced in comparison to normal when there is an increase in lung volume. In diffuse pulmonary fibrosis, the flow rates are normal despite the low lung volumes, the reason for this being that the elastic recoil in these patients is increased. This is a good way of demonstrating how important elastic recoil of the lung is in the generation of airflow.

The CO Transfer Factor

The transfer of CO in the lung is dependent on many physiological variables and for this reason it is a very non-specific test of lung function. Resistance to transfer of CO in the lung is divided into two components.

1. The 'resistance' of the pathway from mouth to pulmonary

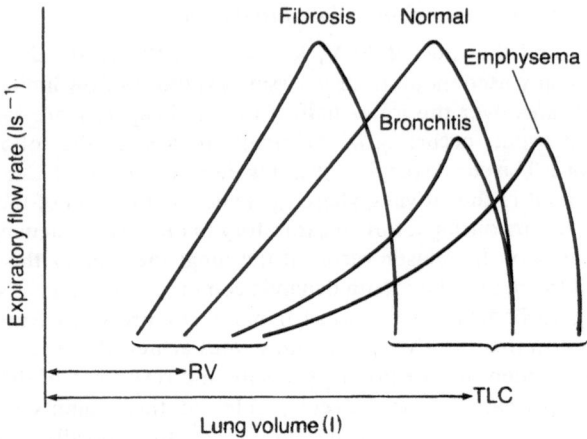

Figure 11. *Flow volume curves in various diseases.*

capillary plasma. This is often referred to by the rather confusing term 'the membrane component'.

2. The uptake of CO by the red cell. This is the red cell component. Roughton and Forster (1957) followed this line of thought to produce the equation:

$$\frac{1}{T_{L}co} = \frac{1}{DM} + \frac{1}{\theta Vc}$$

$T_{L}co$ = transfer factor of the lung for CO; DM = membrane component (alveolus→plasma); θ = number of millilitres of gas taken up by the red cells in one ml of blood/min/mm Hg pressure gradient; Vc = volume of blood in pulmonary capillaries exposed to alveolar gas. The sum of two conductances, A and B, in series must be calculated as follows:

$$\frac{1}{Sum} = \frac{1}{A} + \frac{1}{B}$$

It is possible to calculate the value of the membrane and red cell components. θ, the rate of CO uptake, varies with the oxygen tension. If θ varies, then the $T_L co$ will vary accordingly. By calculating $T_L co$ at two known O_2 tensions, when θ has been calculated for each O_2 tension it is possible to calculate the values of the membrane and red cell components. The values for these two components are about equal, i.e. the 'resistance' to the transfer of CO is equally divided between the 'membrane' component and the red cell component. Variables affecting these two components are given below.

Variables Affecting the Membrane Component

1. The surface area of alveoli available for gas exchange.

2. The correct matching of ventilation and perfusion.

3. The 'resistance' to diffusion of the alveolar cell, the interstitial fluid and the pulmonary capillary endothelium.

Variables Affecting the Red Cell Component

1. The volume of blood in the pulmonary capillaries exposed to alveolar gas. The degree of congestion or distension of the pulmonary capillaries with blood is more important than the time spent by each red cell in contact with the alveoli.

2. The haemoglobin concentration.

3. Rate of uptake of CO with haemoglobin (θ).

Lung Function in Disease

Alteration in lung function as a result of disease is normally divided into two categories: airflow obstruction and a restrictive defect.

Airflow Obstruction

The basic functional abnormality in airflow obstruction is a reduction in the FEV_1, PEFR and the FEV_1/FVC ratio. There are three groups of patients who all have this functional abnormality in common, i.e. patients with asthma, chronic obstructive bronchitis and emphysema. There is often considerable overlap amongst these groups. Lung function testing will help in distinguishing these groups if the following measurements are made:

1. T_Lco and Kco. These measurements are most useful in detecting emphysema. The loss of alveolar membrane and the associated loss of pulmonary capillary vessels reduces gas transfer considerably. The T_Lco will be reduced in asthma and chronic obstructive bronchitis because of poor distribution of the inhaled CO. However, the Kco will be within normal limits whereas it will be low in emphysema.

2. Variability of airflow obstruction. Asthma is usually defined as a disease characterized by wide variations in resistance to flow in intrapulmonary airways over short periods of time. The peak flow meter is the most convenient way of demonstrating this variability by recording the peak flow soon after rising in the morning and then in the evening or during an attack of breathlessness. By comparison, patients with chronic obstructive bronchitis and emphysema vary little in the amount of airflow obstruction.

3. TLC. It is probable that all patients with significant airflow obstruction have an increase in TLC (Gibson and Pride 1976). In emphysema the loss of elastic recoil explains this phenomenon. In asthma and chronic obstructive bronchitis the mechanisms are not so well understood. The largest increase in lung volumes is seen in emphysema and by comparison the increase in TLC in asthma and bronchitis is usually much smaller.

Restrictive Defects

Parenchymal lung disease that results in small, stiff lungs is the commonest type of restrictive pattern seen in clinical practice, e.g. fibrosing alveolitis and sarcoidosis. The TLC is reduced because of an increase in the lung elastic recoil and the FEV_1 and FVC are reduced in proportion so that the forced expiratory ratio is within normal limits. The ratio may even be high as the FEV_1 is relatively well maintained because of the increase in elastic recoil. The transfer factor and Kco are reduced for complex reasons. Loss of surface area of alveoli, impairment of ventilation perfusion ratios and, to a lesser extent, an increase in resistance to diffusion across

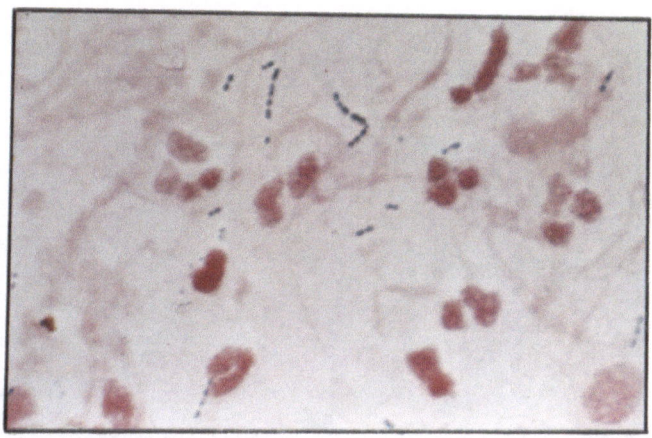

Plate 1. *Sputum. Gram positive cocci from a case of pneumococcal pneumonia.*

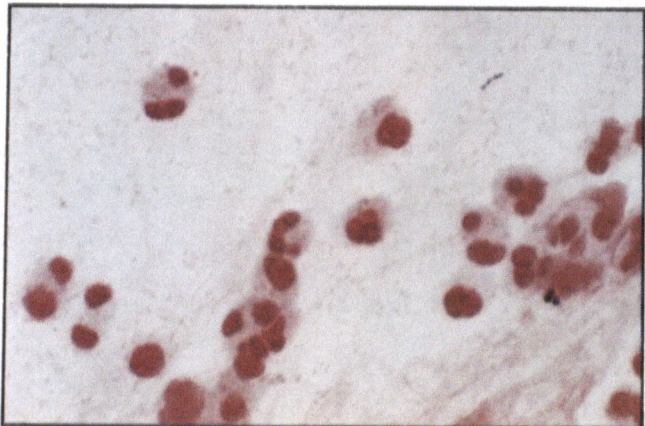

Plate 2. *Sputum. Gram negative cocco-bacilli (*Haemophilus influenzae*) from a patient with an acute exacerbation of chronic bronchitis.*

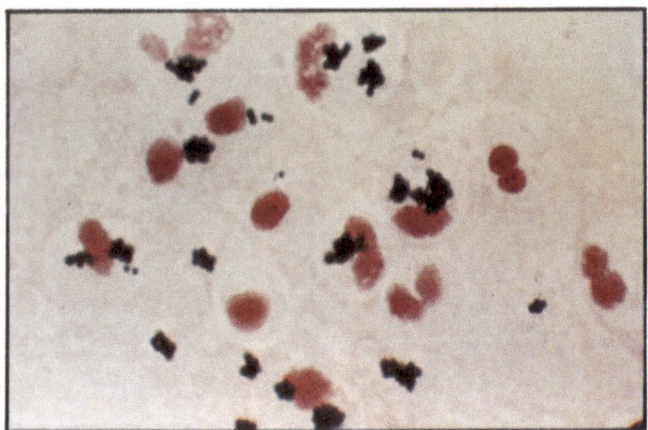

Plate 3. *Sputum. Clusters of Gram positive cocci (many intracellular) from a case of staphylococcal pneumonia.*

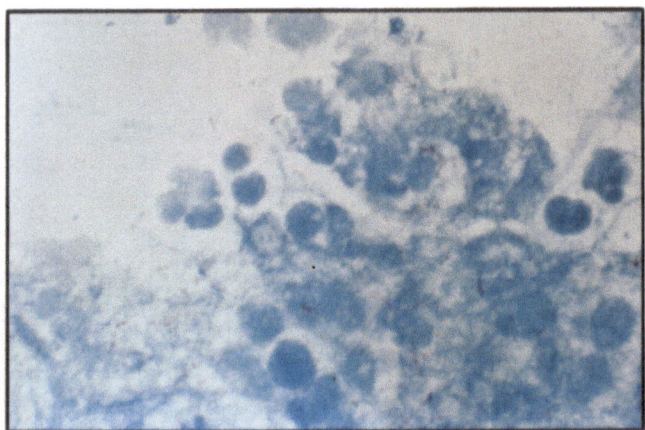

Plate 4. *Ziehl–Nielsen stain: acid fast rods from a case of open tuberculosis.*

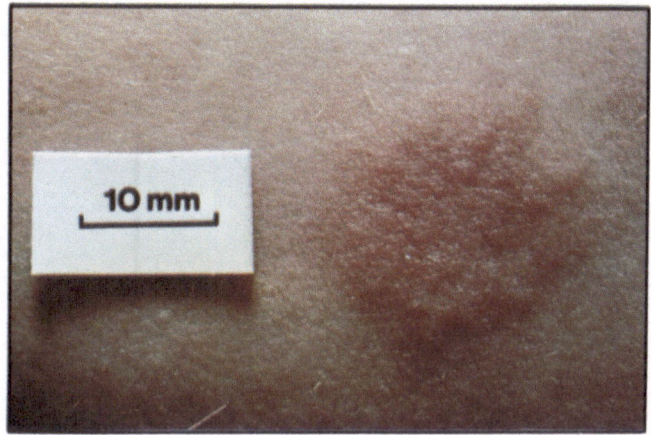

Plate 5. *A positive Mantoux test is a typical type IV hypersensitivity reaction.*

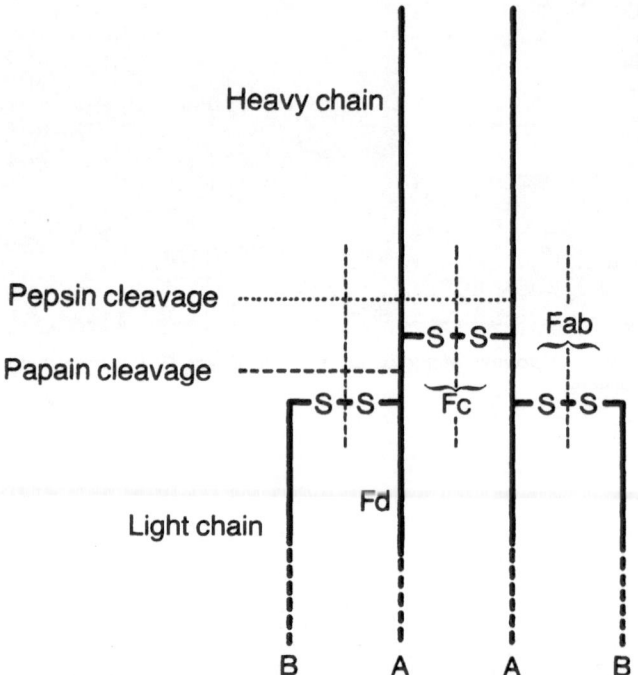

Plate 6. *Immunoglobulin structure (after Porter). Papain cleavage (dashed line) produces two Fab portions and one Fc portion. Pepsin cleavage (dotted line) produces F(ab')X. Disulphide bond reaction produces two light and two heavy chains. The amino acid sequences at the NH₂ terminal (dotted) ends of the chains are variable and form the region carrying specific combining sites.*

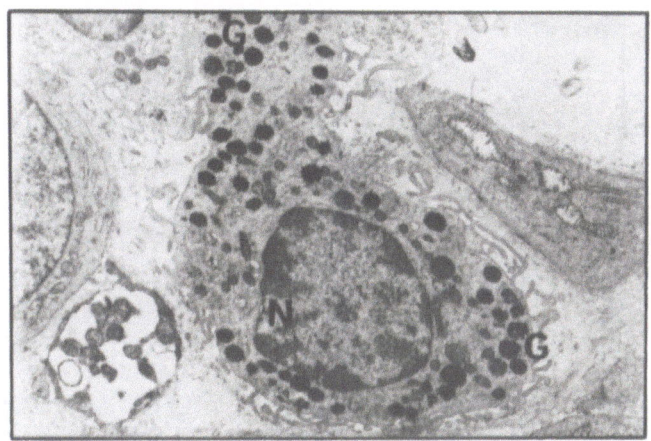

Plate 7. *An electron micrograph of a mast cell from a rat lung (G = granules, N = nucleus).*

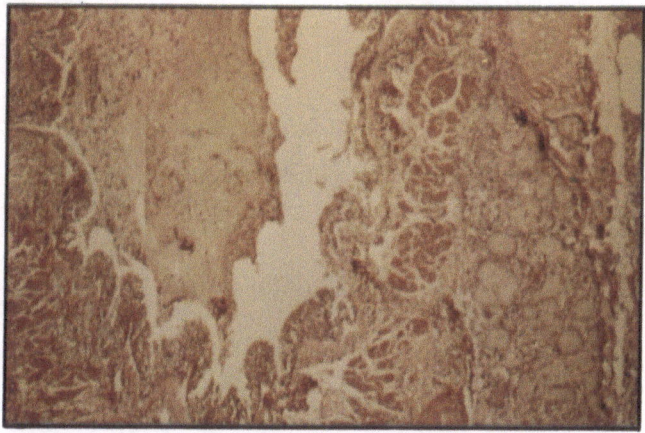

Plate 8. *Section of human lung taken postmortem after fatal status asthmaticus. The lumen of the airway is filled with an amorphous pink staining mucus, there is submucosal oedema with hypertrophy of the peribronchial smooth muscle.*

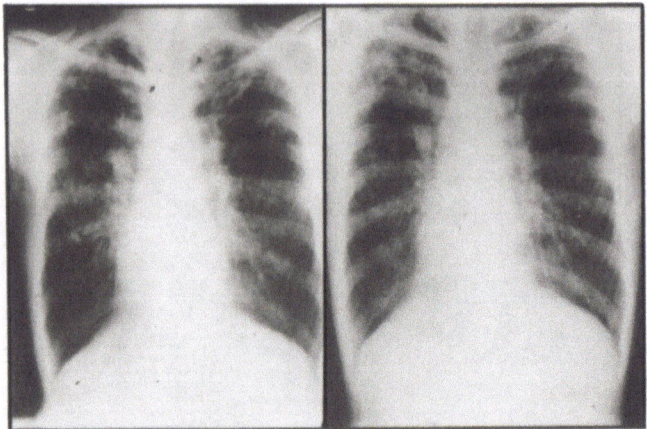

Plate 9. *Patchy transient peripheral lung shadows in a case of bronchopulmonary allergic alveolitis (due in this patient to* Aspergillus fumigatus*).*

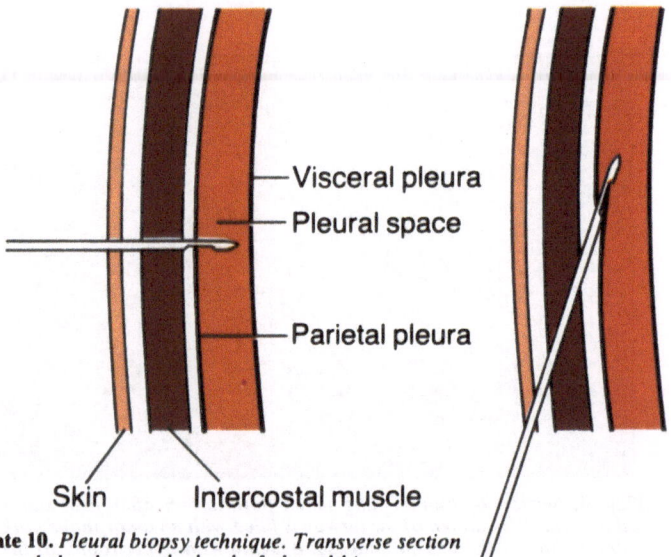

Visceral pleura

Pleural space

Parietal pleura

Skin   Intercostal muscle

Plate 10. *Pleural biopsy technique. Transverse section through the chest at the level of pleural biopsy.*

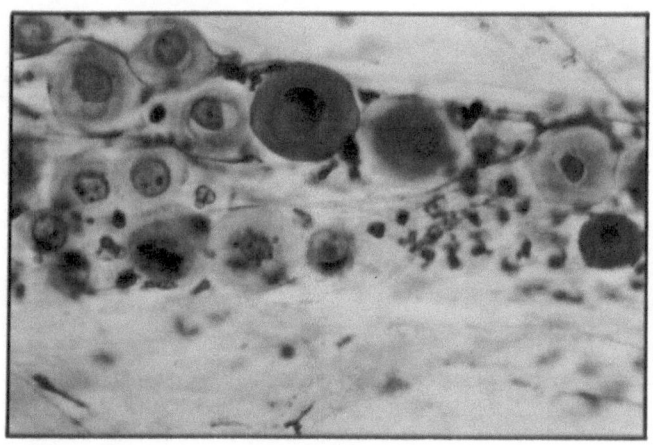

Plate 11. *Malignant keratinized squamous cells.*

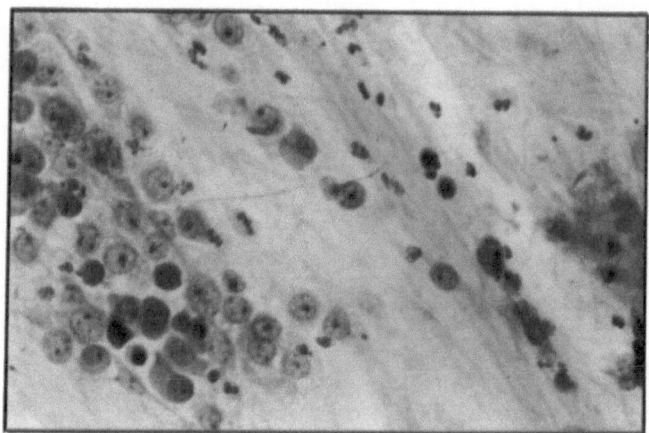

Plate 12. *Sputum. Malignant poorly differentiated squamous cells.*

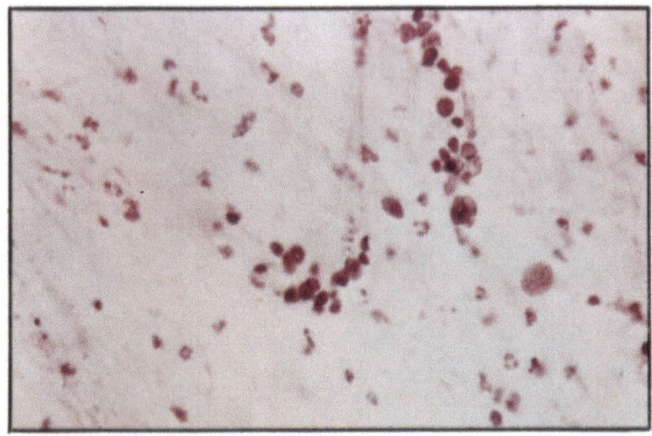

Plate 13. *Sputum. Malignant 'oat cells' (anaplastic small cell carcinoma of bronchus).*

the thickened alveolar membrane are all factors contributing to the loss of gas transfer (McHardy 1972).

Assessing Response to Treatment

The monitoring of the peak flow in patients with airflow obstruction is now well established practice. In diseases which are inherently variable it is of greater value to make a simple measurement, such as the peak flow, on many occasions, rather than more sophisticated measurements on a much smaller number of occasions. In the outpatient clinic measurements taken at each visit are useful, but should be interpreted with greater caution when assessing response to a change in therapy. Continuous twice-daily peak flow measurements, preferably before and after an inhalation of bronchodilator, are the best way of assessing any change in asthmatics' lung function. It is very important to have an adequate control period of measurement before initiating any new therapy, such as corticosteroids. Measurements should continue while the patient is on the new treatment and then be compared with measurements taken during the control period. In

Table 7. Typical changes in lung function tests in various diseases.

	Asthma	Chronic obstructive bronchitis	Emphysema	Fibrosing alveolitis
PEFR	↓	↓	↓	→
FEV_1	↓	↓	↓	↓
FVC	↓	↓	↓	↓
FER	↓	↓	↓	→↑
T_{LCO}	→↓	→↓	↓	↓
VA	↓	→↓	↓	↓
K_{CO}	→↑	→↓	↓	↓
Effect of bronchodilators on PEFR	+ + + greater than 20%	Less than 15%	Less than 15%	No effect

this way it is easier to assess any genuine change in lung function in patients in whom improvement is questionable from the history.

Patients with small, stiff lungs are more stable than patients with airflow obstruction. The relaxed vital capacity and gas transfer are good ways of assessing response to treatment. It is very important to appreciate that single measurements of lung function must be interpreted with great caution because the normal range of values is very large. When lung function tests are reported, predicted values are usually quoted. It should be routine practice to quote the normal range rather than the mean. Table 7 summarizes the typical changes in lung function tests in asthma, chronic obstructive bronchitis, emphysema and fibrosing alveolitis.

5. Arterial Blood Gases and Acid–Base Balance

Arterial Puncture

It is important to obtain the specimen of arterial blood in an atraumatic and airtight fashion. Except in severely hypotensive subjects the taking of arterial blood from the femoral artery is unnecessary and traumatic and will almost certainly lead to alveolar hyperventilation, making the results of the investigation worthless. The ideal site in adults is the radial artery of the non-dominant side, having first determined that the ulnar artery is present. The advantages of using the radial artery are that it is readily palpable, distinct from large veins and can be easily compressed after puncture; haematoma formation is readily apparent and the palmar arch supplies collateral circulation. Local anaesthetic (one per cent plain lignocaine) decreases local pain and, hopefully, any associated hyperventilation.

Arterial blood gases with a $Pa\text{CO}_2$ below 3.3 kPa (25 mm Hg) and a pH greater than 7.47 should alert one to the possibility of alveolar hyperventilation unless the primary pathology could account for such a respiratory alkalosis. Interpretation of $Pa\text{O}_2$ and $Pa\text{CO}_2$ is impossible without knowing the inspired oxygen concentration at the time the sample was taken. Respiratory failure has been classically defined by Campbell (1964) as a $Pa\text{O}_2$ of less than 8.0 kPa (60 mm Hg) and/or a $Pa\text{CO}_2$ greater than 6.65 kPa (50 mm Hg). However, the age of the patient must be considered, as a young man with acute asthma would be thought to have significantly impaired gas exchange with a $Pa\text{O}_2$ of 8.65 kPa (65 mm Hg), although he would not be defined as having respiratory failure.

Principles

Most laboratories when asked for arterial 'blood gases' will measure the partial pressure of oxygen and carbon dioxide and the pH on their respective electrodes. Normal respiration maintains the arterial partial pressure of oxygen (Pao_2) around 13.3 kPa (100 mm Hg), even though oxygen requirements vary from as much as two to three litres/min during strenuous exercise to as little as 100 ml/min during sleep. Alterations in respiration are reflected in changes of the Pao_2 and $Paco_2$ and fall into four main categories. These categories are partially interdependent and pulmonary or other disease may well lead to abnormal blood gases by one or more of the following:

1. Change in alveolar ventilation.

2. Venous to arterial shunting.

3. Impaired diffusion.

4. Mismatching of alveolar ventilation and pulmonary blood flow.

$$\dot{V}_A/\dot{Q} = \frac{\text{Alveolar ventilation per unit time}}{\text{Pulmonary capillary perfusion per unit time}}$$

The Pco_2 is related to the alveolar ventilation, but the Po_2 is a poor indicator of alveolar ventilation because of the different shapes of the CO_2 and O_2 dissociation/association curves. The CO_2 dissociation curve is almost linear (Figure 12) and if alveolar ventilation doubles, the alveolar Pco_2 will halve, the $Paco_2$ will halve and the arterial CO_2 content will fall proportionately. However, the Po_2 in the alveolus will increase above 13 kPa (100 mm Hg) but the increase in O_2 content will be minimal, because the O_2 dissociation curve at this point is nearly horizontal (Figure 13).

If there is hypoventilation, the Pao_2 will fall, but with a correspondingly large fall in oxygen content, again because of the slope of the dissociation curve. A reduced arterial oxygen (Pao_2) with a normal $Paco_2$ is usually associated with 2, 3, 4 (above), or any combination of these. Throughout the normal lung $\dot{V}_A/\dot{Q}$ is unevenly matched and this mismatching is even more pronounced

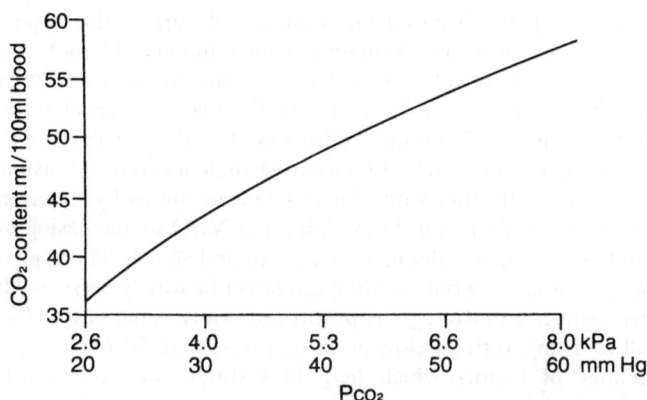

Figure 12. *The CO_2 dissociation curve.*

in the diseased lung, the apex of the lung having a high $\dot{V}_A/\dot{Q}$ and the base a low $\dot{V}_A/\dot{Q}$

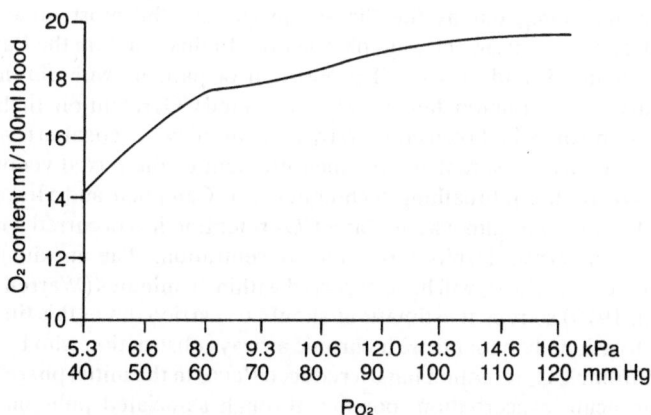

Figure 13. *The O_2 dissociation curve.*

Increasing the inspired O_2 tension will correct the hypoxia during hypoventilation by increasing the number of O_2 molecules present in the alveolus. It will correct the hypoxia due to an alveolar diffusion defect by increasing the alveolar arterial oxygen gradient and so facilitating diffusion. It will also correct the hypoxia due to uneven $\dot{V}_A/\dot{Q}$ since, with high inspired O_2 tensions, those parts of the lung with a high $\dot{V}_A/\dot{Q}$ compensate by increasing the O_2 in solution, and those with a low $\dot{V}_A/\dot{Q}$ by increasing the number of O_2 molecules in poorly ventilated alveoli. The hypoxia due to venous–arterial shunting can never be totally corrected by increasing inspired oxygen concentration and any increase in Pa_{O_2} will be comparatively slow and small (less than 10 per cent). A number of factors which help in distinguishing the various pathophysiological causes of hypoxaemia and carbon dioxide retention are shown in Figure 14.

Clinical Disorders

The commonest pulmonary disorder seen in clinical practice is chronic airways obstruction where the initial defect is associated with small airways obstruction leading to ventilation/perfusion mismatching, but as the disease progresses the most notable defect is increasing airways obstruction. In this situation the Pa_{O_2} is reduced, and in a small proportion of patients with chronic airways obstruction there may be associated CO_2 retention. In this group controlled oxygen therapy is required with repeat arterial blood gas measurements (or measurement of the mixed venous P_{CO_2} by the rebreathing technique—see Campbell and Howell 1962) to ascertain whether any CO_2 retention has occurred with the increased inspired oxygen concentration. The maximum increase in Pa_{CO_2} will have occurred within 30 minutes (Warrell et al. 1970) so repeat estimations should be carried out at this time. Occasionally patients with chronic airways obstruction who have chronic CO_2 retention have a reduced Pa_{CO_2} in the initial phase of an acute exacerbation, possibly through associated pulmonary oedema, which may increase their respiratory drive and therefore 'blow off' their excess CO_2; unless carefully controlled oxygen therapy is used then the patient may be precipitated into CO_2 narcosis.

Other examples of reduced alveolar ventilation are patients who have taken an overdose of a respiratory depressant or patients with myasthenia gravis or Guillain–Barré syndrome affecting the respiratory muscles. In these patients, who are usually young with normal gas exchange mechanisms, arterial blood gas measurements are of only secondary importance. By the time there is a significant fall in Pao_2 the minute volume and tidal volume are greatly reduced, and the patient's requirement for ventilatory support should be decided upon these measurements rather than arterial blood gas estimations. Ideally on admission Pco_2 and $Paco_2$ should be related to ventilation, as this will give some indication of the patient's gas exchange.

In patients with neuromuscular disease the vital capacity is the best index of ventilation, and if the vital capacity falls below two litres, ventilatory support is usually required (Pontopiddan 1972).

Impaired diffusion is seen classically in fibrosing alveolitis and pulmonary oedema and is associated with a reduction both in Pao_2 and $Paco_2$. Venous to arterial shunting can be from either cardiac or intrapulmonary lesions and is a severe example of $\dot{V}_A/\dot{Q}$ mismatching. This is seen with pneumonia and more recently has been identified as a major problem in the 'shock lung' or adult respiratory distress syndrome. This occurs in a number of conditions in which the patient is severely ill, and is associated with a loss of vital capacity, increasing lung stiffness with a rapid respiratory rate and severe hypoxaemia. There is usually an initial fall in $Paco_2$ associated with the increased respiratory drive from compliance changes of the lung, but if the patient deteriorates the $Paco_2$ may rise to normal or higher and unless ventilatory support is instituted it may lead to death.

Acute pulmonary embolism is usually associated with an initial fall in Pao_2 with a reduced $Paco_2$ and a respiratory alkalosis. However, in moderate pulmonary embolism the Pao_2 may rise to the normal range quite rapidly, so a normal Pao_2 does not exclude this diagnosis, especially in the presence of a respiratory alkalosis.

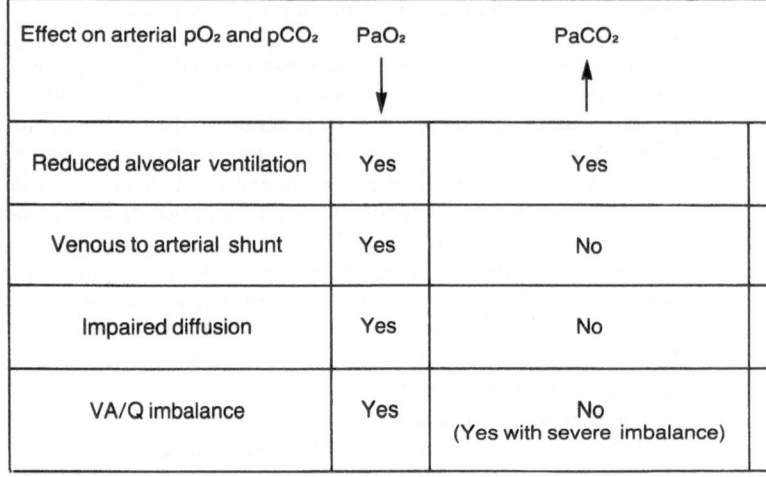

Effect on arterial pO_2 and pCO_2	PaO_2 ↓	$PaCO_2$ ↑
Reduced alveolar ventilation	Yes	Yes
Venous to arterial shunt	Yes	No
Impaired diffusion	Yes	No
VA/Q imbalance	Yes	No (Yes with severe imbalance)

Figure 14. *Features helpful in distinguishing the various causes of hypox-aemia and carbon dioxide retention.*

Acid–Base Balance

Metabolic processes produce acid in the form of carbon dioxide, which generates carbonic acid, and non-volatile acids. The lungs excrete about 13,000 mmol/day of 'acid' in the form of CO_2 and the kidney excretes about 40 to 80 mmol/day of acid in the non-volatile form. The majority of hydrogen ion in the body is bound to buffer base and only a very small concentration exists as the free hydrogen ion, about 40 nmol/l. These buffer bases are anions which are distributed throughout the body and comprise mainly bicarbonate, protein, haemoglobin and phosphate.

To describe acid–base status it is generally agreed that three values are required: the hydrogen ion concentration, the Pco_2 and the available buffer base. The Pco_2 reflects alveolar ventilation and so is a measure of the respiratory component of acid excretion. Unfortunately there is no easy way of measuring the total

PaO₂ on exercise ↓	PaCO₂ on exercise ↑	Added inspired O₂
Often severe	Severe	Increase in PaO₂
Yes	Occasionally	Slow and small rise in PaO₂
Often severe	No	Increase in PaO₂
Yes	No (Yes with severe imbalance)	Increase in PaO₂

buffer base and usually only part of the buffer base, in the form of HCO_3^-, is measured. It is hoped that this reflects total body buffer base. The total body buffer is a reflection of the non-volatile acid component.

The law of mass action states:

$$K = \frac{[H^+][HCO_3^-]}{[H_2CO_3]}$$

$$[H^+] = \frac{K \times P_{CO_2} \times S}{[HCO_3^-]}, \text{ where } S \text{ is } CO_2 \text{ solubility coefficient.}$$

If the $[H^+]$ and P_{CO_2} are known, then the $[HCO_3^-]$ can be calculated provided that the two constants K and S are known. Although values for these 'constants' are known, they are not in fact constant (Howarth 1974).

Standard Bicarbonate

Since change in the P_{CO_2} will itself change the $[HCO_3^-]$, the concept of equilibrating blood in vitro with a P_{CO_2} of 5.3 kPa (40 mm Hg) was introduced to eliminate the respiratory component and so reflect the non-respiratory (metabolic) component (Jørgenson and Astrup 1957).

Whole Blood Buffer Base

It is possible to measure the whole blood buffer base by titrating blood in vitro with a strong acid and its value is about 45 to 50 mmol/l. The amount of base will vary with the amount of fixed acid but not with the P_{CO_2} and so will reflect the non-respiratory (metabolic) acid–base status. The reason the P_{CO_2} does not affect the total base is that for every HCO_3^- ion generated one of the other base anions (Hb^-, protein$^-$, or phosphate$^-$) will gain an H^+ and become an acid. In the presence of a known Hb^- concentration the buffer base and base excess or deficit relative to normal values can be calculated from nomograms such as the Siggard–Anderson nomograms.

The basic problem with both standard bicarbonate and buffer base is that they are based on in vitro tests on blood and do not reflect what happens in the interstitial fluid and the intracellular fluid. It has been calculated that up to 97 per cent of buffering in the body is done by the intracellular fluid and so it is easy to see the inherent danger of taking the base deficit/excess too literally and attempting to correct an acid–base disturbance based on these results. The relationship between $[HCO_3^-]$, $[H^+]$ and P_{CO_2} in vivo in various acid–base disturbances is now quite well established (Bone et al. 1974; Stoker et al. 1975).

Disorders of Acid–Base Balance

Disorders of acid–base balance are classically divided into respiratory and non-respiratory acidosis and alkalosis. The term metabolic is widely used but imprecise, since respiratory disorders are related to inappropriate excretion or retention of 'metabolically' produced CO_2. We will therefore use the terms 'respiratory' and non-respiratory acidosis and alkalosis.

Non-respiratory Acidosis

In this condition the $[H^+]$ increases and the Paco$_2$ decreases as a result of increased respiratory drive. The primary change is an increase in $[H^+]$, whether this increased $[H^+]$ is from ingestion of acids (e.g. aspirin overdose), from diabetic ketoacidosis where an excess of $[H^+]$ is produced, or from renal failure when there is $[H^+]$ retention. From the law of mass action equation the $[HCO_3^-]$ will decrease, as will the concentration of the other bases which are not measured; they bind $[H^+]$ in an attempt to stabilize the hydrogen ion concentration.

The hydrogen is normally actively secreted by the kidney against a considerable H^+ concentration gradient in exchange for the HCO_3^-. The rate of H^+ secretion is also dependent on the Pco$_2$, secretion increasing with a high Pco$_2$. Thus in non-respiratory acidosis the H^+ secretion by the kidney may tend to fall, because the Pco$_2$ is low and the HCO_3^- available for reabsorption is lowered. However, this decrease in H^+ secretion is compensated by a greater increase in the production of ammonia by the renal tubular cells and this combines with H^+ in the tubular fluid and so reduces the H^+ gradient. Thus the acidosis is partially corrected by the kidneys.

Treatment of this condition involves identifying and correcting the cause and correcting dehydration and electrolyte loss. It is not usually necessary to give $NaHCO_3$ unless the acidosis is very severe. Kassirer (1974) suggests the following formula for the amount of HCO_3^- in mmol:

$$HCO_3^- = \text{body weight (kg)} \times 0.5 \times \text{desired increment in } [HCO_3^-].$$

The rise in serum $[HCO_3^-]$ after therapy based on this simple equation is highly unpredictable and depends on the primary pathology. Acid–base status should be monitored every two to three hours during treatment. It may be dangerous to give HCO_3^- solution, especially by rapid infusion, for several reasons. Posner and Plum (1967) showed that the level of consciousness correlated very well with cerebrospinal fluid (CSF) [H^+] and very poorly with serum [H^+]. In respiratory acidosis, CSF [H^+] increased more than in a comparable non-respiratory acidosis, for reasons not entirely understood, with the result that level of consciousness was better maintained in non-respiratory acidosis. In some of their patients with non-respiratory acidosis given HCO_3^- solutions the previously alert patients become drowsy and they showed that despite a return to normal of the serum [H^+] there was a paradoxical increase in the CSF [H^+]. The hypothesis put forward to explain this was that the improvement in serum acid–base status was in some way responsible for the decrease in hyperventilation, the P_{aCO_2} increased in these patients and so the highly diffusible CO_2 molecule diffused rapidly into the CSF with a resultant increase in CSF [H^+].

Non-respiratory Alkalosis

Non-respiratory alkalosis is uncommon and when severe is usually associated with loss of acid from the stomach as a result of prolonged vomiting. The [H^+] falls and the buffer systems compensate by dissociating buffer acid to form H^+ and increase in buffer base, which is reflected by a high [HCO_3^-] and considerable base excess. The respiratory compensation, although rare clinically, does exist. In the absence of significant respiratory disease the relationship between [H^+] and P_{CO_2} is indirect and curvilinear, the [H^+] decreasing as the P_{CO_2} rises (Bone et al. 1974).

For reasons that are not understood the kidney is partially responsible for the generation and maintenance of non-respiratory alkalosis. The kidneys usually continue to produce an acid urine (paradoxical aciduria). The increase in P_{aCO_2} stimulates H^+ secretion and hence HCO_3^- reabsorption. There is often associated dehydration, hypokalaemia and hypochloraemia, which all contribute to increased hydrogen ion excretion (Seldin and Rector 1972).

Treatment should be directed to replacement of fluid and electrolytes and this is usually all that will be required.

Respiratory Acidosis

The primary fault lies in the respiratory system and CO_2 retention occurs because the lungs are unable to excrete the CO_2 produced by metabolism. CO_2 accumulates and H_2CO_3 is formed which dissociates (at body $[H^+]$) almost completely to H^+ and HCO_3^-. In acute respiratory acidosis the $[HCO_3^-]$ increases by only a few mmol. It is sometimes thought that increasing the P_{CO_2} must increase the HCO_3^- proportionately, but this does not occur because by increasing the P_{CO_2} acutely to 7.5 kPa (60 mm Hg) the increase in the number of CO_2 molecules added to the dissolved CO_2–carbonic acid–HCO_3 system is small in relation to the total number of molecules in this system. Renal compensation does not reach a maximum until a few days after the onset of the acidosis. The H^+ excretion increases secondarily to the increase in the P_{CO_2} and so the reabsorption of HCO_3^- will increase. This increased reabsorption of HCO_3^- causes the large increase in serum HCO_3^- seen in patients with chronic CO_2 retention and is associated with an increase in total body base leading to a base excess.

Respiratory Alkalosis

Acute respiratory alkalosis is caused by alveolar hyperventilation with a resultant fall in P_{CO_2}. H^+ and HCO_3^- associate, which results in a fall in $[H^+]$ and a fall of $[HCO_3^-]$ of a few mmol, analogous to the small rise in $[HCO_3^-]$ during acute respiratory acidosis. During chronic respiratory alkalosis, the kidney excretes less acid than usual which results in less HCO_3^- reabsorption and so the serum $[HCO_3^-]$ falls to levels of approximately 12 to 15 mmol/l with a P_{CO_2} of about 2.6 kPa (20 mm Hg).

Difficulties in Diagnosis

Problems arise in interpretation of acid–base data when the clinician fails to take the patient's history and physical signs into account. By the time blood gas measurements are taken the primary disturbance may or may not have been compensated for by a renal mechanism in the case of primary respiratory disturbance and vice versa. Figure 15 is a rather over-simplified diagram that starts from point A (normal) and goes to the four primary disturbances of acid–base balance, points B, C, D, E. These four primary disturbances, when compensated, go to points H and F. It is oversimplified because the compensatory mechanisms often do not return the $[H^+]$ to normal. Another problem is encountered in cases in which there is a primary respiratory disturbance which is then corrected. The lungs are fast excretors and the kidneys are

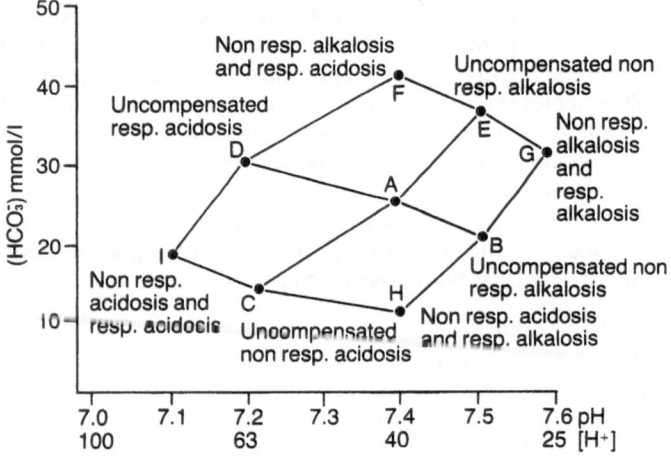

Figure 15. *See text for details.*

slow excretors of acid and in the case of corrected primary respiratory disturbances it takes the kidneys a few hours or even days to catch up. A good example of this was reported by Robin (1963) in patients with chronic lung disease with CO_2 retention. A number of these patients were in the alkalaemic range of $[H^+]$. One of the contributing factors is thought to be the relative improvement in airflow obstruction which occurs from day to day in patients with chronic lung disease. Their P_{CO_2} falls and the $[HCO_3^-]$ remains the same and thus the $[H^+]$ will fall. Another factor that slows the base $[HCO_3^-]$ component correction is the relatively free diffusibility of the CO_2 molecule in comparison to the bicarbonate ion. In Figure 15 this is represented by a move from the primary pathology at point D to the compensated situation at point F and then on to point E. The same problem arises in chronic respiratory alkalosis, point B, which moves to point H and then on to point C if the primary cause for the hyperventilation is removed ('posthypocapnic non-respiratory acidosis'). The commonest clinical situation in which this occurs is in patients who have been on a mechanical ventilator and have been hyperventilated. When allowed to breathe spontaneously they become acidotic and hyperventilate, i.e. move from point B back to point H.

It is essential, however, to realize that arterial blood gas estimation can never be considered in isolation but must be related to the patient's history, physical signs and other investigations. If a therapeutic decision is to be based on the blood gas results, such as giving added oxygen or artificial ventilation, it is essential to know whether the changes are acute or chronic.

6. Immunology and the Lung

The lung is susceptible to all four types of hypersensitivity reactions of the classification of Gell and Coombs. Type I reactions due to interaction between an external allergen and antibodies of the IgE ('reaginic') type are manifested as allergic asthma. Type II or 'cytotoxic' reactions are uncommon, and an example of this type of reaction is that seen in Goodpasture's syndrome where antibodies are directed against alveolar basement membrane. Type III or 'Arthus' reactions are common and result from the production of antibody directed (usually) against an inhaled antigen and the ensuing reaction produces a delayed hypersensitivity alveolitis, typified by 'farmer's lung'. Type IV 'cell-mediated' reactions primarily involve T lymphocytes and, following sensitization, interaction between the sensitized T cells and the antigen results in the formation of granulomas. The tuberculous granulomas resulting from sensitization to the cell wall constituents of *Mycobacterium tuberculosis* is one such type IV reaction. The Kveim reaction obtained in patients with sarcoidosis, and the Heaf skin reaction in tuberculosis, are further examples of type IV reactions (Plate 5). In this chapter we shall be chiefly concerned with types I and III hypersensitivity reactions.

Type I Allergic Lung Disease

The clinical manifestation of type I allergic reactions in the lung is asthma, a common disorder which may vary in severity from mild, occasional wheezing to potentially catastrophic status asthmaticus. In Europe asthma is the sixth commonest cause of non-accidental death among children. The pathological sequence of events in the genesis of allergic asthma is as follows. First, the individual requires some genetic predisposition to respond to an antigenic stimulus by producing IgE antibodies. This genetic factor is known to be important from clinical observation, though in some allergic asthmatics it may not be apparent. In a study of 'atopic' or allergic patients a genetic factor existed in 86 per cent where at least one parent had a similar type I allergic disorder.

The allergic process is initiated following exposure to an antigen (sometimes called an 'allergen'), most often by inhalation of a dust or aerosol of the substance. Circulating B lymphocytes differentiate into IgE-producing plasma cells. The IgE produced in response to this challenge, like all classes of antibody, is a Y-shaped molecule (Plate 6), having a portion which can become attached to a cell surface (the Fc zone) forming the tail of the 'Y'. Each of the arms terminates in a portion which can attach to the antigen (the Fab zone). The Fab zone is specific for the antigen which stimulated its production by the plasma cell and thus confers uniqueness on the antibody.

IgE, whose Fab portions are specific for and directed against one allergen, will react only with that allergen and not with any other. Thus an individual who is allergic to ragweed pollen is not affected by grass pollen or tree pollen. Ragweed-IgE is specific only for ragweed and not for anything else. The IgE thus produced becomes attached by its Fc zone to the outer surface of circulating basophils and to mast cells in the mucous membranes of the airways. These cells contain quantities of potent biologically active substances including histamine, bradykinin and SRS-A ('Slow reacting substance of anaphylaxis') (see Plate 7).

When a mast cell coated with IgE is re-exposed to the allergen for which the IgE is specific, the cytoplasmic granules of bioactive amines are secreted into the surrounding tissues. It is these mast cell granules which mediate the acute reaction, producing spasm of bronchial smooth muscle, increased capillary permeability leading to local oedema of the airways mucosa and increased production of thick, tenacious mucus. This triad of events leads to narrowing or occlusion of the airways (see Plate 8). It is important to appreciate that the pathology of asthma is thus not simply bronchospasm since both this and to some extent the mucosal oedema may be relieved by bronchodilator drugs, theophyllinates and steroids. The mucous plugs occluding the already narrowed lumen of the air passages are less amenable to drug treatment and are a major cause of failure of treatment and of death.

The role of eosinophils in the acute type I reaction is uncertain. They are frequently found in the peripheral blood, lung tissue and sputum of patients with asthma but are not peculiar to allergic asthma, since they are also present in the type of asthma designated 'intrinsic' in which no allergen-IgE reaction can be demonstrated. One role which they appear to play is the secretion of a chemical factor which inhibits the renewal of the mast cell granules. They also secrete histaminase and aryl sulfatase, enzymes which deactivate histamine and SRS-A, respectively.

The blood, tissue and sputum eosinophilia is abolished quite quickly by systemic steroid therapy, the blood eosinophils being the first to disappear, usually within a few hours of starting treatment, and the sputum eosinophilia disappears within two to four days. Presumably eosinophils migrate from the circulation into the pulmonary tissue, and thence into the airways and are then expectorated in the sputum.

Prick testing consists of applying one drop of a special liquid extract of the suspected or potential allergen to the volar aspect of the forearm and pricking it gently through the epidermis (not the full skin thickness) with the point of a small hypodermic needle or lancet. Studies have shown that the results of prick tests correlate well with both nasal and bronchial provocation tests so that these latter can be reserved for patients where there is a strong index of suspicion of an allergic aetiology to their asthma and the results of skin tests are equivocal—probably less than five per cent of cases. It is emphasized, however, that one must not treat the results of prick tests but use them as an adjunct to a careful history.

Type III Allergic Lung Disease

Type III allergic alveolitis differs in several respects from type I. In type I reactions, described above, the principal antibody involved is IgE, in type III reactions it is IgG. There is some evidence that some type I reactions may be mediated by short-term IgG antibodies but they are of doubtful significance.

In type III allergic lung disease IgG antibodies are produced in response to inhaled antigens—usually after prolonged and heavy exposure. The reaction is not acute but delayed for about six hours after exposure. It is characterized clinically by cough, dyspnoea, fever and general malaise. There is a raised erythrocyte sedimentation rate, and an acute inflammatory infiltration in the lung parenchyma, with peripheral polymorphonuclear leucocytosis and raised eosinophil count. The infiltration is seen on the chest radiograph as patchy shadowing (Plate 9), the extent of which matches the degree of exposure and severity of the illness. The patchy shadows are transient and resolve as the reaction subsides.

Some authorities report that granulomas similar to those seen in type IV reactions may also be a feature of allergic alveolitis, suggesting that there may be a cell-mediated component to the reaction. Repeated attacks of alveolitis may lead to irreversible damage with fibrosis as the end-stage, in contrast to type I reactions where irreversible damage does not occur. Examination of the blood will show the presence of precipitating IgG antibodies directed against the antigen, and will also show that the reaction involves complement consumption. Type III alveolitis is not as common as type I allergic asthma, generally because the degree and length of exposure to the antigen needs to be greater.

Typically the type III alveolitis occurs in an otherwise non-atopic (i.e. non-allergic) person, and in some illnesses such as farmer's lung where the antigen is the spores of the mould *Micropolyspora faeni*, which grows on rotting hay, both IgG and IgE antibodies may be produced, resulting in a dual reaction. There is then an immediate type I allergic asthma, and a delayed type III alveolitis, with a positive prick test and circulating precipitins. Farmer's lung is not confined to farmers: their cows also contract the disorder, then known as 'fog-fever', if fed on mouldy hay. Both farmers and cattle develop the disease in the late winter months when fresh fodder is scarce and the previous year's mouldy hay is being used for feed and bedding.

Less common fungal allergic alveolitides include 'mushroom picker's lung' in which the spores responsible are those of *Thermoactinomyces sacchari*, and 'malt-whisky distiller's lung' occurs in about five per cent of men engaged in the malt whisky distilling industry. When the malt germinates the men may be exposed to huge amounts of *Aspergillus clavatus* spores.

There are now many types of allergic alveolitis described which are peculiar and specific to the industrial process in which the patients affected are engaged—baker's asthma, hairdresser's asthma, meat-wrapper's asthma, bagassosis, bird-fancier's lung, etc. However, byssinosis, one of the most common causes of industriál lung disease caused by the inhalation of organic dust, is not immunologically mediated but closely simulates allergic asthma. Byssinosis consists of bronchoconstriction caused by a chemical of high molecular weight found in the bracts of the cotton plant; this chemical causes mast cells to release mediators spontaneously.

The Mycetoma

A mycetoma is a ball of fungus growing in a lung cavity produced by some other disease process—usually a tuberculous cavity. In a series of 544 patients with healed tuberculous cavities, 11 per cent had mycetomas. Very often the radiographic appearances alone are strongly indicative of the diagnosis and serological examination will reveal precipitins as found in allergic alveolitis. Thus some diagnostic confusion may arise between an acute alveolitis due to, for example, *Aspergillus fumigatus* and an aspergilloma. Since the latter may be expectorated usually with haemoptysis, both diseases fulfil the diagnostic criteria of transient lung shadows with circulating precipitins. However, the antigenic stimulus from the presence of a thriving mycelium growing in a cavity is very great and on immunodiffusion the patient's serum will show many more precipitin arcs than are found in allergic aspergillosis of the type III alveolitis.

7. Invasive Investigations in Lung Disease

Pleural Fluid Aspiration

Pleural fluid aspiration is used in the diagnosis of some lung diseases and also as a therapeutic manoeuvre to relieve dyspnoea. The pleural fluid obtained for diagnostic purposes should be examined for the following:

1. The macroscopic appearance may be clear with a light yellow colour ranging through various shades of yellow to a massively blood-stained effusion. Blood-stained effusions are very often secondary to a neoplasm involving the pleura. Exudates have a varying number of cells present and, if left to stand, will clot. Transudates are clear and watery and often bilateral. Purulent fluid from an empyema is usually self-evident and a large diameter needle or drainage catheter may be required to remove all the pus if it is very dense. Chylous effusions are milky in appearance and are usually secondary to surgical trauma or neoplastic invasion of an intrathoracic lymph duct.

2. Cytology is helpful in differentiating a tuberculous effusion from an acute bacterial postpneumonia effusion, lymphocytes being present in the former and polymorphs in the latter. Cytology for the presence of malignant cells requires expert interpretation before a confident diagnosis can be made.

3. Bacteriology of pleural fluid should be carried out on all the fluid remaining after a sample has been set aside for biochemistry. The fluid can be spun and the sediment cultured. In this way the yield, particularly in tuberculous effusions, will be improved.

4. Biochemistry should include a protein concentration determination if differentiation between a transudate and exudate is required. A protein concentration of 30 g/l suggests an exudate, but serum protein should also be estimated. The glucose concentration in pleural effusion secondary to rheumatoid arthritis is often low (<1 mmol/l). Lactic dehydrogenase levels are raised in patients with pleural effusions associated with rheumatoid arthritis.

Pleural Biopsy

Pleural biopsy, using an Abrams needle, is very useful provided the operator is experienced. Many doctors obtain either no pleura or inadequate specimens because of an improper technique. The 'notch' on the needle should be facing downwards while in the pleural space, the needle is then withdrawn and the notch will engage the pleura, intercostal muscle and possibly rib. The needle is then rotated through 90° and will now contain pleura and intercostal muscle but no possibility of rib. The needle will have been at 90° to the chest wall throughout the procedure so far. The needle is now pushed in such a way that its length comes to lie tangentially to the chest wall (Plate 10) while *maintaining the same depth*, and the specimen is then taken in the usual way. This last manoeuvre increases the likelihood of obtaining pleura.

Thoracoscopy

Thoracoscopy is a useful technique in which a cannula is introduced into the pleural space followed by a telescope, a direct inspection of the visceral and parietal pleura can be performed with an accompanying biopsy. It is possible to instil a substance (e.g. iodized talc) that will cause an inflammatory response of the pleural surfaces and so promote pleural adhesion if it is felt that the appearances at thoracoscopy are due to malignant infiltration of the pleura. It is therefore possible in some cases to perform aspiration, make a histological diagnosis and perform palliative treatment in one manoeuvre.

Bronchoscopy

The most important indication for bronchoscopy is the search for evidence of lung cancer. The advent of fibreoptic bronchoscopy has been a major advance in the management of chest disease. It has two distinct advantages over the rigid bronchoscope. It is much easier to pass into the bronchial tree and it has a greater visual and biopsy range than the rigid bronchoscope. The rigid bronchoscope is still the method of choice for removal of foreign bodies. The positive bronchial biopsy rate in lung cancer using the rigid bronchoscope is in the region of 50 per cent and using the fibreoptic bronchoscope (FOB) is about 70 per cent. Collection of specimens for bacteriology via the bronchoscope is very unrewarding (see Chapter 3), except in the case of tuberculosis, where lavage and subsequent aspiration of contents from the upper lobes in suspected tuberculosis may reveal *Mycobacterium tuberculosis*.

Lung Biopsy

Lung tissue can be obtained via the airways, a transbronchial biopsy (TBB), or directly through the chest wall by needle or drill.

Transbronchial Biopsy

Flexible forceps are passed out into a peripheral bronchus until resistance is met. The patient is then asked to inhale, the forceps are opened; the patient exhales fully and the forceps are closed. During exhalation bronchial and pulmonary tissue are pushed into the jaws of the forceps. The forceps are withdrawn and a good specimen of lung tissue is usually obtained.

Brush Biopsy

Brush biopsy involves passing a nylon brush on the end of a flexible steel guide wire out into an abnormal area via a FOB, either under direct vision onto an endobronchial lesion or into an abnormal area of lung using an image intensifier for guidance. This technique is less traumatic than forceps biopsy, but has the big disadvantage of only providing material for cytology. The skill of the cytologist is probably the single most important factor in the success rate of brush biopsy techniques.

Percutaneous Needle and Drill Biopsy

This technique has been developed to include a range of needles varying from very fine aspiration needles to cutting needles such as the trucut needle and the air drill driven cutting needle. The samples obtained from aspiration needles vary considerably depending on the type of lung tissue sampled, normal lung and dense lesions often providing an inadequate tissue. The trucut cutting needle provides larger specimens of lung tissue and is better able to penetrate dense lung lesions such as diffuse fibrosing alveolitis.

Complications

Pneumothorax is a common complication, but the majority require no treatment. Haemoptysis is the most dangerous complication and needle biopsy in the presence of pulmonary hypertension or any form of bleeding disorder is more likely to cause haemoptysis.

Open Lung Biopsy

Open lung biopsy is a technique that provides sufficient lung tissue for a diagnosis to be made in the majority of cases. Gaensler et al. (1964) had a 95 per cent positive biopsy rate in 105 patients who underwent open biopsy.

Conclusions

TBB is safer than other methods of lung biopsy and is easily performed at the end of a routine fibreoptic bronchoscopy. The biggest single disadvantage is that the size of the biopsy is too small to be of use in many diffuse lung diseases. In those patients with malignant disease and a normal FOB it should be possible to prove a diagnosis of malignancy by TBB in approximately 60 to 70 per cent. Patients who are immunocompromised and/or uraemic, presenting with abnormal shadowing on the chest radiograph will also benefit from TBB since lung tissue demonstrating intracellular organisms or malignant tissue may be obtained. Aspiration needle biopsy is of value in suspected malignant disease when TBB has revealed no results and a diagnosis is required without resorting to thoracotomy. The needle biopsy, particularly with small peripheral lesions, is more accurate than TBB, lesions as small as 1 cm in diameter being amenable to biopsy. In nonmalignant lesions needle biopsy is likely to provide more useful information than TBB because the size of biopsy is greater. However, in diffuse lung disease the tissue is often inadequate for good histology. Drill biopsy is not as commonly used as needle aspiration biopsy and TBB. In patients with diffuse lung disease such as fibrosing alveolitis, and the pneumoconioses open lung biopsy is frequently required before a definitive diagnosis can be made.

8. Diagnostic Cytology

Cytology is a valuable technique in the diagnosis of suspected carcinoma of the bronchus, although it is too expensive a procedure for routine screening in the same way as cervical cytology.

There are four methods of obtaining material for examination: sputum, bronchial brush biopsy, saline washing of the bronchi and fine needle aspiration.

Sputum

Sputum can be expected to be positive in about 60 per cent of cases. Three specimens should be collected from the patient on consecutive days, and the specimens should be taken first thing in the morning. The specimens must be sputum, as saliva is useless. Each specimen should reach the cytology laboratory as soon as possible. If six specimens are negative, further examination should only be performed in selected cases, as only a small return in terms of positive results can be expected for considerable expenditure of time (Plates 11, 12 and 13).

Bronchial Brush Biopsy

When a tumour cannot be visualized or biopsied on bronchoscopy, bronchial brushing performed through a fibreoptic bronchoscope with fluoroscopic control if necessary, is the technique of choice.

The positive results rate for brushing is about 70 per cent, and if this investigation is preceded by sputum examination, the combined rate is about 90 per cent.

Saline Washing of the Bronchi

Saline washing of the bronchi via a fibreoptic bronchoscope is an alternative to the brush technique. The percentage of positive results obtained with this technique is about the same as that obtained with the brush method. Immediate cytological examination is again essential.

Fine Needle Aspiration

For peripheral lesions visualized on the chest radiograph, fine needle aspiration is a useful method for obtaining cytology material. Malignant cells may be present in sputum for months, even years, before a tumour can be visualized on a straight radiograph. It is important to localize the lesion as early as possible, when it is still treatable. Some tumours occur in a scarred part of the lung where growth is very slow, and others are diagnosed at a very early stage.

Well differentiated carcinomas and small cell anaplastic carcinomas (oat cell) can be typed accurately by cytology. The incidence of false positives should be very low with this method. However, difficulties can arise with squamous metaplasia and dysplasia, bronchiectasis, old cavities and fungal infections.

9. Perfusion and Ventilation Lung Scanning

As in many other branches of respiratory medicine, the use of radionuclides to image the different functions of the lung is a recent development. The clinical application of these techniques began following the work of Wagner in 1963 who used a single intravenous injection of microparticles labelled with a gamma-ray emitting radionuclide and was able to diagnose pulmonary emboli accurately without the need for an invasive procedure. Improvements in the imaging equipment, with the introduction of the gamma-camera by Anger in 1968, have made it possible to view the different surfaces of the lung, providing the facility of defining the anatomy of functional defects. Finally, with the provision of the newer gaseous radionuclides obtained from a cyclotron, e.g. the short half-life krypton-81m, defects of ventilation may also now be visualized.

Techniques

The great advantage of lung scanning is that it provides a non-invasive method of viewing the principal functions of the lung: ventilation and perfusion.

The perfusion image is obtained by a single intravenous injection of microparticles made from human albumin (either microspheres or macroaggregates), which are labelled with technetium 99 m ($^{99}Tc^m$). These microparticles exhibit two important characteristics: a similar density to red blood cells, and a range in size between 10 and 70 μm. The similar density to red blood cells, following mixing in the right ventricle, enables the distribution of the microparticles within the lung to be in proportion to the regional pulmonary blood flow. The size range results in their being temporarily obstructed within a tiny proportion of the 300 million pulmonary arterioles which range in size between 15 and 30 μm in diameter. As a result of this, the gamma-ray emitting ^{99}Tc^m is concentrated in proportion to the regional pulmonary blood flow within the pulmonary arterioles.

A comparable ventilation image may be obtained using krypton-81m, which has a half-life of 13 seconds. This inert gaseous radionuclide is obtained by air elution from a generator containing the parent isotope rubidium-81m. The resulting air–^{81}Kr^m mixture is breathed quietly by the patient, and when a steady state is achieved the concentration of the ^{81}Kr^m within the distal airspaces is proportional to the regional alveolar ventilation. A further advantage of the use of the combination of ^{99}Tc^m and ^{81}Kr^m is that their gamma ray emissions are at different energy levels (141 and 190 Kev, respectively). Using a variable energy 'window' on the gamma-camera, successive perfusion and ventilation images of the same view of the lung can be obtained without repositioning the patient in front of the camera.

To obtain each perfusion and ventilation image requires only minimal co-operation from the patient, who must simply remain positioned in front of the gamma-camera (see Figure 16) for a period of three to six minutes for each view . It is usual to obtain six views of the perfusion of the lungs: anterior, posterior, right and left laterals, and right and left posterior oblique. Ventilation images are usually obtained for those views where disturbances of regional perfusion are most prominent, so that an exact comparison can be made between the anatomical distribution of the perfusion and ventilation defects.

Clinical Application

Pulmonary Embolic Disease

The principal clinical role of lung scanning is in the diagnosis of pulmonary embolism. Pulmonary emboli produce a wide spec-

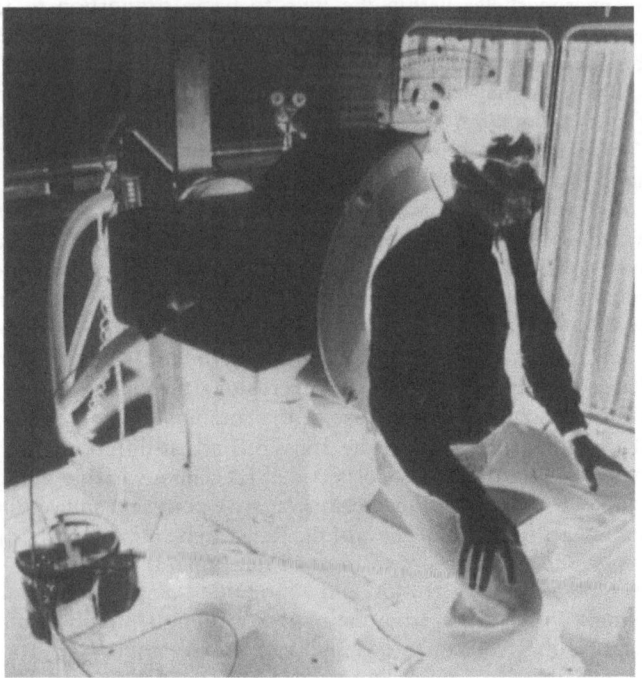

Figure 16. *The patient may sit or lie in front of the wide view gamma camera breathing via an MC mask the air–krypton–81m gas mixture. The injection of microspheres or macroaggregates labelled with technetium 99m having been performed earlier. A fan placed behind the camera directs any free krypton–81m away from the camera. The different views of the lung are obtained by simply rotating the patient in front of the camera.*

trum of clinical presentations from the 'silent' small emboli to the massive, invariably fatal, emboli, where over 50 per cent of the pulmonary circulation is obstructed. Diagnostically, the clinician is interested in one question—whether or not to anticoagulate the patient as prophylaxis against further emboli, often in patients where there is suspicion alone of pulmonary embolism. The lung scan is particularly suited to answering such a question. It is a non-invasive procedure requiring little patient co-operation and it provides as accurate a diagnosis of pulmonary emboli as pulmonary arteriography. Two aspects of pulmonary embolic disease lend themselves to the use of lung scanning. First, emboli from the venous system frequently result in obstruction of the segmental pulmonary arteries producing a picture of multiple anatomical segmental defects. Second, these segmental perfusion defects are *not* associated with comparable defects in ventilation. These are believed to be due to the weakness in man of bronchoconstriction which has been seen in animals after pulmonary arterial obstruction, and to the prevalence of collateral ventilation of lobar segments in man. This mismatching between perfusion defects and ventilation produces characteristic lung scans in pulmonary emboli.

Examples of Pulmonary Emboli

The first example is of a 32-year-old man who developed rapidly progressive glomerular nephritis and who was treated with corticosteroids. Six months after the onset of his kidney disease he developed exertional dyspnoea. Physical examination revealed no abnormalities and he had a normal chest radiograph (see Figure 17) and a normal electrocardiogram. As a result of a high index of suspicion a lung scan was performed which revealed bilateral segmental perfusion defects (these were clearly seen on the left and right posterior oblique and posterior views of the lung, see Figures 18, 19 and 20). This picture alone is characteristic of pulmonary embolic disease, but was further confirmed by the absence of similar segmental ventilation defects (see Figure 21 for the posterior view of the lungs ventilation).

The second example is of a woman of 45 years who, more typically for pulmonary embolic disease, presented with a pleuritic right-sided chest pain and haemoptysis two weeks post-operatively. Again there were no abnormal physical signs to be found on examination but her chest radiograph revealed a right-sided upper zone shadow and pleural effusion (see Figure 22). Bilateral perfusion defects were seen on the lung scan (see Figures 23 and 25 for anterior and posterior views). The ventilation images, however, revealed no such abnormalities (Figures 24 and 26).

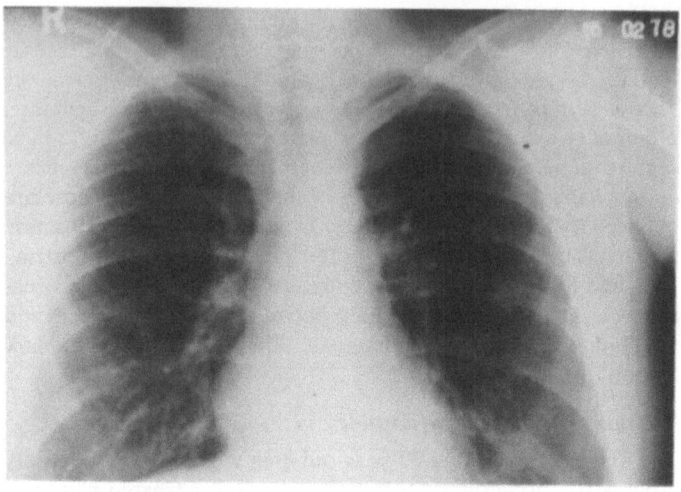

Figure 17. *The chest radiograph of a 32-year-old man with glomerular nephritis, who developed dyspnoea.*

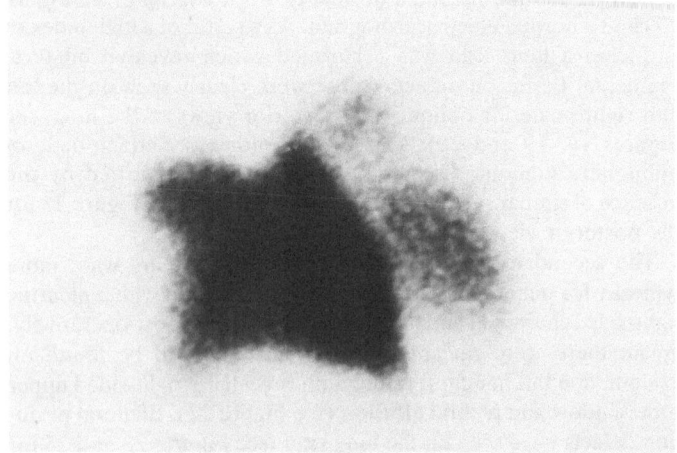

Figure 18a. *The left posterior oblique view of the perfusion image of the patient in Figure 17, showing the segmental defects.*

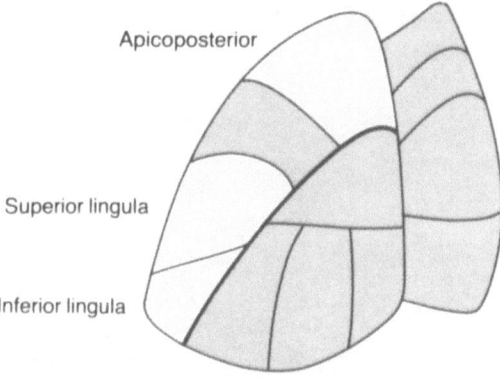

Left posterior oblique

Figure 18b. *A schematic drawing of the same view as in Figure 18a, with the segmental structure of the lung revealing the defects in the apicoposterior and lingular segments of the left lung.*

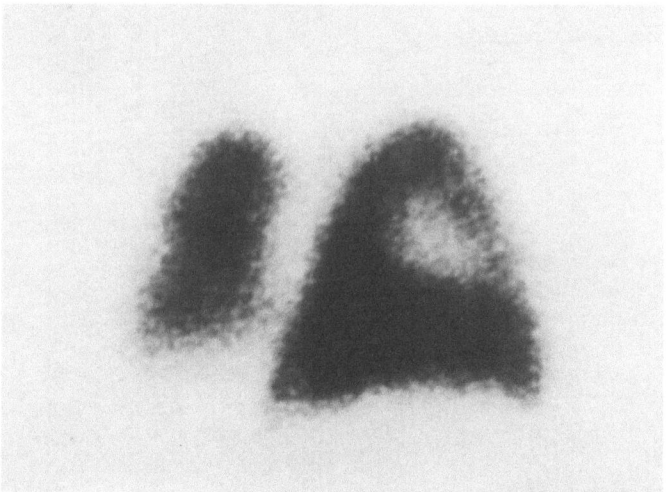

Figure 19a. *The right posterior oblique view of his perfusion image.*

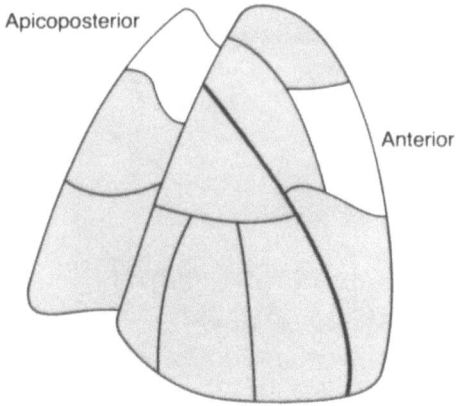

Right posterior oblique

Figure 19b. *The schematic segmental structure of the same views of the lung showing a partial anterior segmental defect on the right and apicoposterior defect on the left.*

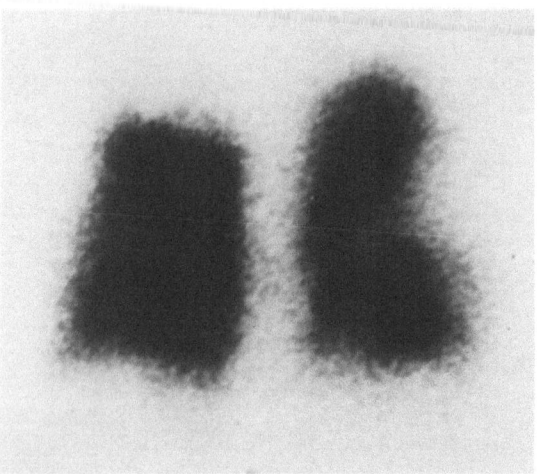

Figure 20a. *The posterior perfusion image of the lungs with the bilateral defects shown.*

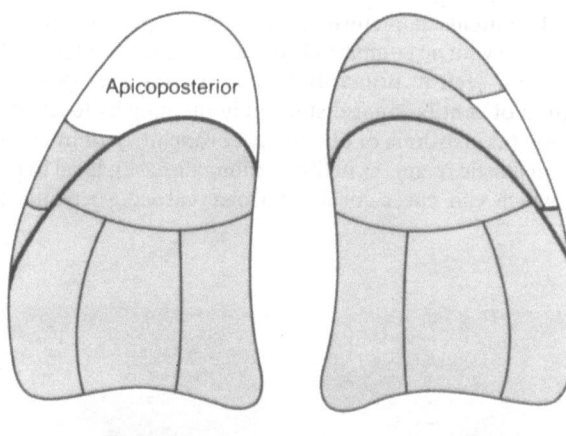

Figure 20b. *The segmental structure of the posterior views of the lung showing the left apicoposterior and right anterior defects.*

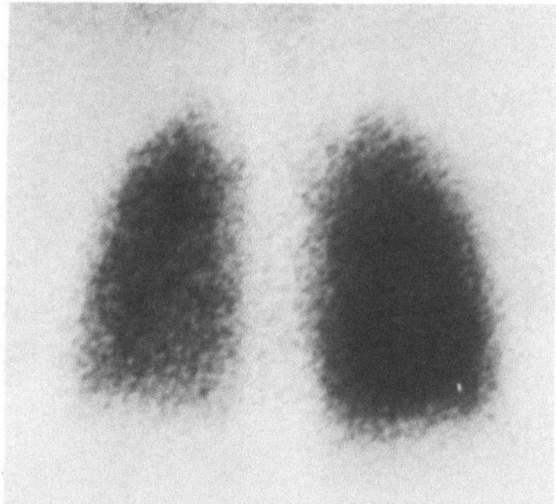

Figure 21. *The posterior ventilation image showing the normal distribution of ventilation with no segmental defects.*

In both patients a picture of multiple segmental perfusion defects is seen with no comparable disturbance of ventilation. This pattern is not seen in primarily lung-based diseases. When the distribution of ventilation is disturbed in the lung by local airway obstruction (as in asthma or obstructive bronchitis), or by changes in the local elastic recoil (as in fibrotic lung disease), local hypoxia results, which can cause local arteriolar vasoconstriction. This

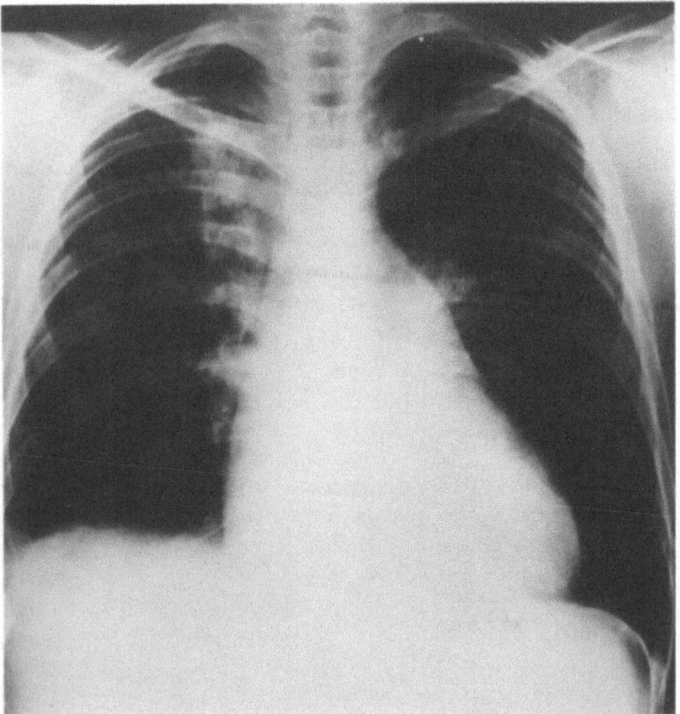

Figure 22. *The chest radiograph of a 45-year-old woman showing a right upper zone shadow with a small right-sided pleural effusion and fluid in the horizontal fissure. A prominent pulmonary conus can be seen.*

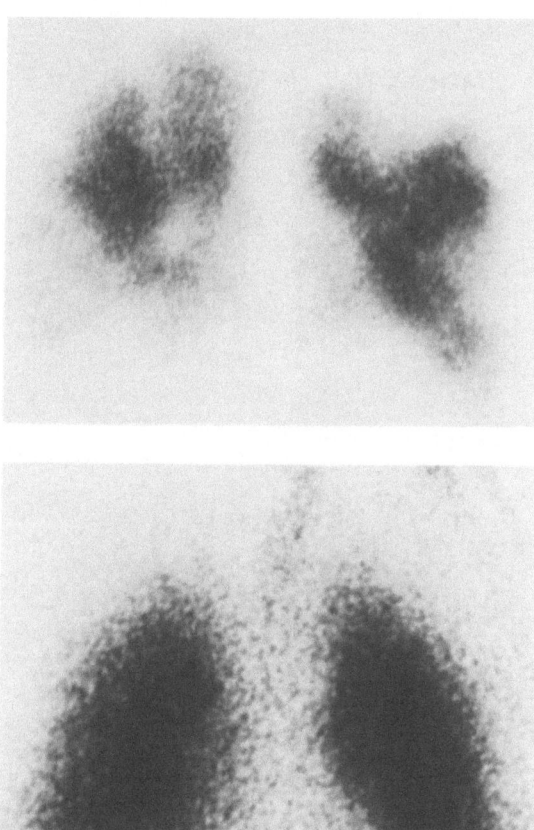

Figures 23 and 24. *The anterior views of the ventilation and perfusion images from the same patient as in Figure 22 with the multiple bilateral perfusion defects but a normal ventilation image.*

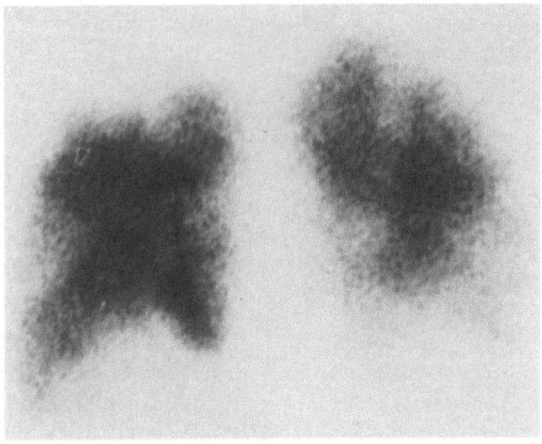

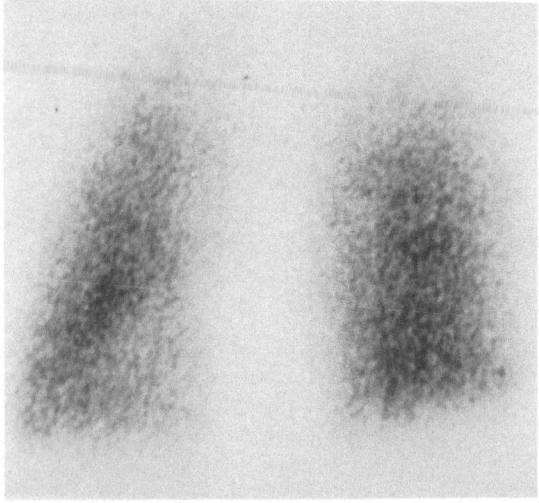

Figures 25 and 26. *The posterior perfusion and ventilation images of the same patient showing again the multiple bilateral defects with almost normal ventilation image. Note the straight right lower border to the ventilation image representing the right pleural effusion.*

represents part of the pulmonary homeostatic mechanism which enables a balance between ventilation and perfusion to be maintained and produces a characteristic perfusion and ventilation image in which defects in both modalities appear matched.

Examples of Chronic Obstructive Bronchitis

A 48-year-old woman who had suffered from wheezing, breathlessness and a productive cough since childhood was studied. Clinically she had bilateral wheezes on auscultation, and her forced expiratory volume in one second (FEV_1) was only 25 per cent of the predicted value. The chest radiograph revealed hyperinflated lung fields but no lung shadow (see Figure 27). Despite this, both the perfusion and ventilation images of her lungs revealed widespread matching defects (see Figures 28 and 29 for the posterior views of the perfusion and ventilation images). The same sort of matching between perfusion and ventilation defects is seen in many primary lung diseases and heart failure.

Problems in Diagnosis of Pulmonary Emboli

Scans

Despite the clear qualitative difference between the perfusion and ventilation lung images produced by pulmonary emboli and other primary lung disease there may remain two areas of interpretive difficulties:

1. Embolic obstruction of the pulmonary arteries is only short-lived. In people younger than 65 years who have no coexisting pulmonary and cardiovascular disease the emboli 'disintegrate' and pass distally, finally leaving no trace over a period of between seven days and three months. It is possible to miss single or multiple embolic pulmonary arterial obstruction, if the perfusion scan is not performed close enough to the presentation of the disease.

2. In patients with coexisting lung disease, pulmonary infarction with haemorrhage into the alveoli may occur, due to the paucity of

the bronchial circulation which normally retains the viability of
segments of the lung in which their pulmonary arteries have
become obstructed by emboli. As a result there will be matching
perfusion and ventilation defects in this situation. Thus, although

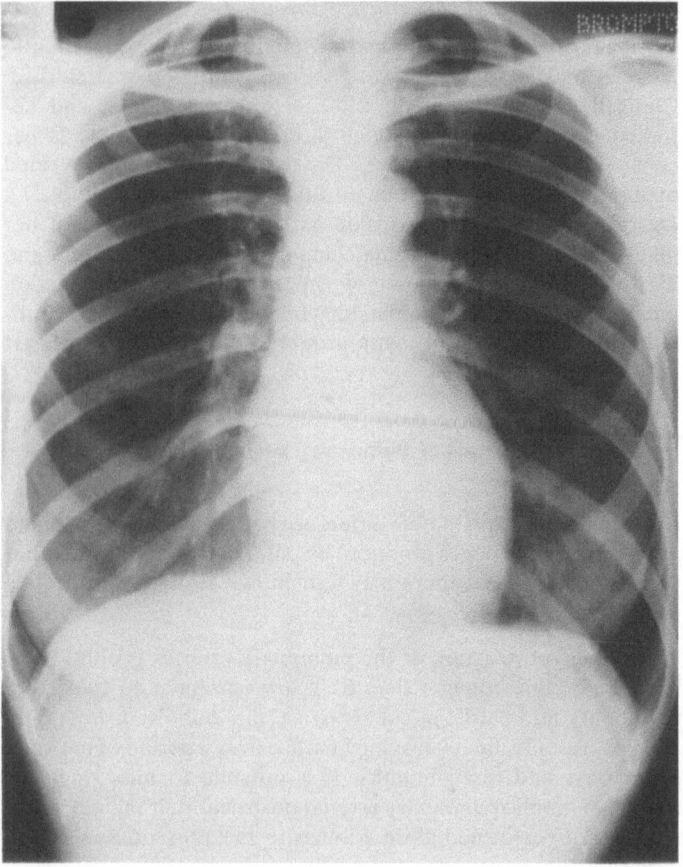

Figure 27. *The hyperinflated lung fields of a chronic obstructive bronchitic
woman on whom the vascular markings in the left upper and midzone
probably reflect an element of emphysema.*

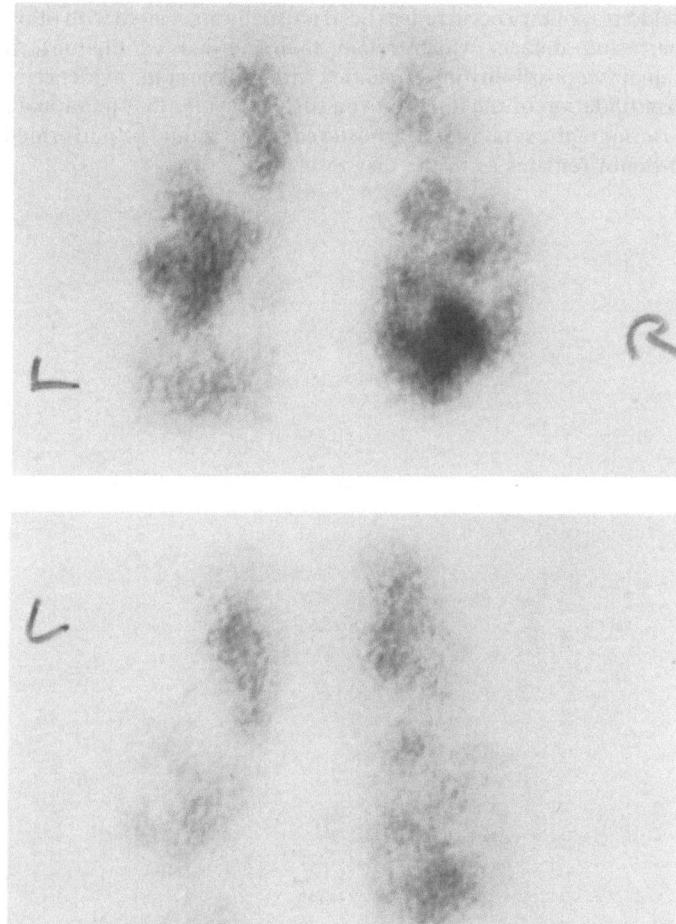

Figures 28 and 29. *The posterior perfusion and ventilation images respectively from the woman with chronic airflow obstruction with the largely matching ventilation and perfusion defects.*

seldom a solitary occurrence (i.e. it is usually associated with other perfusion defects which retain their normal ventilation), it remains a possibility in all patients with radiographic evidence of consolidation of the lung. It is on such occasions that pulmonary arteriography retains its diagnostic edge and should be performed if doubt remains as to the diagnosis.

References

Chapter 1

Doll, R. and Hill, A. B., *Br. Med. J.*, 1964, **1**, 1399.

Hampton, J. R., Harrison, M. J. G., Mitchell, J. R. A., Prichard, J. S. and Seymour, C., *Br. Med. J.*, 1975, **2**, 486.

Johnson, R. N., Lockhart, W., Ritchey, R. T. and Smith, D. H., *Br. Med. J.*, 1960, **1**, 592.

Poole, G. and Stradling, P., *Br. Med. J.*, 1964, **1**, 341.

Chapter 2

Boyd, D., *Br. J. Dis. Chest*, 1975, **69**, 259.

Forgacs, P., *Lung Sounds*, Baillière Tindall, London, 1978.

Nath, A. R. and Capel, L. H., *Thorax*, 1974, **29**, 223.

Chapter 4

Dubois, A. B., Botecho, S. Y., Bedell, G. M., Marshall, R. and Comroe, J. H., *J. Clin. Invest*, 1956, **35**, 322.

Forster, R. E., Cohn, J. E., Briscoe, W. A., Blakemore, W. J. and Riley, R. L., *J. Clin. Invest*, 1955, **34**, 1417.

Fry, D. and Hyatt, R. E., *Am. J. Med.*, 1960, **29**, 672.

Gibson, G. J. and Pride, N. B., *Br. J. Dis. Chest*, 1976, **70**, 143.

Hutchinson, J., *Med. Chir. Trans.*, 1846, **29**, 137.

McHardy, G. J. R., *Br. J. Dis. Chest*, 1972, **66**, 1.

Peress, L., Sybrecht, G. and Macklem, P. T., *Am. J. Med.*, 1976, **61**, 165.

Pride, N. B., *Br. J. Dis. Chest*, 1971, **65**, 135.

Roughton, F. G. W. and Forster, R. E., *J. Appl. Physiol.*, 1957, **11**, 290.

Chapter 5

Bone, J. M., Cowie, J., Lambie, A. T. and Robson, J. S., *Clin. Sci. Molec. Med.*, 1974, **46**, 113.

Campbell, E. J. M., *Br. Med. J.*, 1964, **2**, 1328.

Campbell, E. J. M. and Howell, J. B. L., *Br. Med. J.*, 1962, **2**, 630.

Howarth, P. J. N., *Lancet*, 1974, **i**, 253.

Jørgenson, K. and Astrup, P., *Scand. J. Clin. Lab. Invest.*, 1957, **9**, 122.

Kassirer, J. P., *N. Engl. J. Med.*, 1974, Oct. 10, 773.

Pontopiddan, C., *New. Engl. J. Med.*, 1972, **287**, 743.

Posner, J. B. and Plum, F., *New. Engl. J. Med.*, 1967, **277**, 605.

Robin, E., *New. Engl. J. Med.*, 1963, **268**, 917.

Seldin, D. W. and Rector, F. C., *Kidney Internat.*, 1972, **1**, 306.

Stoker, J. B., Kappagoda, C. J., Snow, H. M. and Linden, R. J., *Clin. Sci. Molec. Med.*, 1975, **48**, 133.

Warrell, D. A., Edwards, R. M. T., Godfrey, S. and Jones, N. L., *Br. Med. J.*, 1970, **2**, 252.

Chapter 7

Gaensler, E. A., Moister, M. V. B. and Hamm, J., *New Engl. J. Med.*, 1964, **270**, 1319.

Further Reading

Chapter 2

Lillington, G. A. and Jamplis, R. W., *A Diagnostic Approach to Chest Disease: Differential Diagnoses based on Roentgenographic Patterns*, Williams and Wilkins, Baltimore, 1977.

Simon, G., *Principles of Chest X-ray Diagnosis* (3rd ed.), Butterworths, London, 1972.

Chapter 3

Bartlett, R. C., *Medical Microbiology—Quality Cost and Clinical Relevance*, John Wiley and Sons, Bristol, 1974.

El-Regaie, M. and Dulake, C., *J. Clin. Path.*, 1975, **28**, 801.

Freeman, R., *Infection and Intensive Care in Selected Topics in Clinical Bacteriology*, J. de Louvois (Ed.), Baillière Tindall, London, 1976.

Gardner, P. S. and McQuillin, J., *Rapid Virus Diagnosis, Applications of Immunofluorescence*, Butterworths, London, 1974.

Murray, P. R. and Washington, J. A., *Mayo Clin. Proc.*, 1975, **50**, 339.

Thorsteinsson, S. B., Musher, D. M. and Fagan, T., *J. Am. Med. Assoc.*, 1975, **233**, 894.

Wilson, M. J. B. and Martin, D. E., *J. Clin. Path.*, 1972, **25**, 697.

Chapter 6

Citron, K. M., *Proc. R. Soc. Med.*, 1975, **68**, 587.

Gell, P. G. H., Coombs, R. P. A. and Lachman, P. T., *Clinical Aspects of Immunology*, Blackwell Scientific, Oxford, 1975.

Roitt, I. M., *Essentials of Immunology*, Blackwell Scientific, Oxford, 1977.

Chapter 8

Zajicek, J. and Karger, S., *Aspiration biopsy cytology*, Monographs in Clinical Cytology, Part 1, Basel, London, 1974.

Chapter 9

Fazio, F. and Jones, T., *Br. Med. J.*, 1975, **3**, 675.

Wagner, H. N., Jr., *Am. Rev. Resp. Dis.*, 1976, **113**, 203.

Yono, Y., McRae, J. and Anger, H. O., *J. Nuc. Med.*, 1970, **11**, 674.

Index